Diversity, Inclusion and Culture Wars in Psychotherapy

For the psychotherapist/psychological therapist, notions of diversity and inclusion, such as intersectional feminist, trans*, critical race/whiteness, migration, (in)equality, queer, disability, post-colonial, decolonial, approaches and studies, are both increasingly important and yet increasingly difficult. This book explores these developments and raises the important questions: Are these difficulties to do with the biases of the person who is the psychotherapist, and/or could it also sometimes have to do with how diversity, inclusion and related terms are constructed?

Crucially, clients may now find it difficult to find a therapist who is able to explore with them their concerns around diversity and inclusion which can be complicated and may take time to consider. This book presents cutting-edge research to enable explorations of our changing world which is so different to the one we were born into (let alone our, often older, own psychotherapists and supervisors).

Diversity, Inclusion and Culture Wars in Psychotherapy will be a beneficial read for students and scholars of Psychology including Psychotherapy and Counselling. The chapters in this book were originally published as a special issue of *European Journal of Psychotherapy and Counselling.*

Del Loewenthal is Emeritus Professor of Psychotherapy and Counselling at the University of Roehampton and is Chair of the Southern Association for Psychotherapy and Counselling (SAFPAC), London, UK. He is an existential-analytic psychotherapist and a chartered psychologist, with a particular interest in phenomenology. His books include *Existential Psychotherapy and Counselling after Postmodernism* (2017). www.delloewenthal.com; www.safpac.co.uk

Diversity, Inclusion and Culture Wars in Psychotherapy

Edited by
Del Loewenthal

Routledge
Taylor & Francis Group
LONDON AND NEW YORK

First published 2024
by Routledge
4 Park Square, Milton Park, Abingdon, Oxon, OX14 4RN

and by Routledge
605 Third Avenue, New York, NY 10158

Routledge is an imprint of the Taylor & Francis Group, an informa business

British Library Cataloguing-in-Publication Data
A catalogue record for this book is available from the British Library

ISBN13: 978-1-032-69546-4 (hbk)
ISBN13: 978-1-032-69548-8 (pbk)
ISBN13: 978-1-032-69550-1 (ebk)

DOI: 10.4324/9781032695501

Typeset in Minion Pro
by codeMantra

Publisher's Note
The publisher accepts responsibility for any inconsistencies that may have arisen during the conversion of this book from journal articles to book chapters, namely the inclusion of journal terminology.

Contents

Citation Information

The following chapters were originally published in the *European Journal of Psychotherapy and Counselling*, volume 25, issue 1–2 (2023). When citing this material, please use the original page numbering for each article, as follows:

Chapter 1
Queer minds, Queer needs
Erene Hadjiioannou and Julian-Pascal Saadi
European Journal of Psychotherapy and Counselling, volume 25, issue 1–2 (2023), pp. 12–28

Chapter 2
Therapy and diversity – an (un)therapeutic relationship?
James M. Sedgwick
European Journal of Psychotherapy and Counselling, volume 25, issue 1–2 (2023), pp. 29–43

Chapter 3
A psychotherapist's lived experience in-session with an asylum seeker and translator: An autoethnographic case study
Nicole Chew-Helbig
European Journal of Psychotherapy and Counselling, volume 25, issue 1–2 (2023), pp. 44–59

Chapter 4
Being seen: The lived experience of psychodynamic practitioners disclosing or not disclosing sight impairment
Laura Evers
European Journal of Psychotherapy and Counselling, volume 25, issue 1–2 (2023), pp. 60–88

Chapter 5
How might psychotherapy improve its service to disabled people and people with physical impairment?
Sally Parsloe

European Journal of Psychotherapy and Counselling, volume 25, issue 1–2 (2023), pp. 89–101

Chapter 6
Towards an integrative model of multicultural responsiveness
Daryl Mahon
European Journal of Psychotherapy and Counselling, volume 25, issue 1–2 (2023), pp. 102–126

Chapter 7
Deconstructing humanitarian compassion: Ψ as method
Artemis Christinaki
European Journal of Psychotherapy and Counselling, volume 25, issue 1–2 (2023), pp. 127–144

Chapter 8
Diversity and aggression: A reflection on sensual meanings and an ameliorative law after Freud and Lacan
Tony McSherry
European Journal of Psychotherapy and Counselling, volume 25, issue 1–2 (2023), pp. 145–158

Chapter 9
An exploration of lesbian and gay people's experiences of religion, and their implications for psychotherapy: An Interpretative Phenomenological Analysis (IPA)
Peter Meades
European Journal of Psychotherapy and Counselling, volume 25, issue 1–2 (2023), pp. 159–178

Chapter 10
Contemporary psychotherapy: Evolution in our modern time
Silva Neves
European Journal of Psychotherapy and Counselling, volume 25, issue 1–2 (2023), pp. 179–197

Chapter 11
Diversity in counselling & psychotherapy
Gillian Proctor
European Journal of Psychotherapy and Counselling, volume 25, issue 1–2 (2023), pp. 198–209

Notes on Contributors

Nicole Chew-Helbig is a gestalt psychotherapist currently in private practice based in Singapore. She is currently pursuing a doctorate in Psychotherapy Science in Sigmund Freud University, Vienna, Austria.

Artemis Christinaki is Lecturer in Global Health in the Humanitarian and Conflict Response Institute (HCRI) at the University of Manchester, UK. His PhD research critically explores what are the politics or, the role of, psycho-social support in the refugee camps of Greece. It focuses chiefly on the way aid workers' subjectivities emerge amid the spatial temporality of camps and within the combined discourses of psychology and aid.

Laura Evers has an MSt. in Psychodynamic Practice from Oxford University, UK. She is a psychodynamic postgraduate course tutor at Oxford University, therapist and supervisor in private practice. She qualified in 2014 and has previous experience working in the secondary and tertiary education sectors counselling students, accredited by UKCP.

Erene Hadjiioannou is an integrative psychotherapist offering psychotherapy, training, speaking and writing services via her private practice in Leeds. Her focus is on supporting survivors of sexual violence of any gender. Knowing that the mental health system is largely inaccessible to many, including when it intersects with legal systems, Erene acts on her social responsibility as a psychotherapist. In particular, she is part of an independent steering group working to change the Crown Prosecution Service guidelines on pre-trial therapy and engages in activism and community support.

Del Loewenthal is Emeritus Professor of Psychotherapy and Counselling at the University of Roehampton and is Chair of the Southern Association for Psychotherapy and Counselling (SAFPAC), London, UK. He is an existential-analytic psychotherapist and a chartered psychologist, with a particular interest in phenomenology. His books include *Existential Psychotherapy and Counselling after Postmodernism* (2017). www.delloewenthal.com; www.safpac.co.uk

Daryl Mahon is a psychotherapist, lecturer and researcher. Prior to taking up his current role in research Daryl worked across the social inclusion sector, working with individuals and communities facing marginalisation. Much of his work has centred on substance use with people who also involved in the criminal justice system, mental health difficulties and homelessness. Daryl also lectures in Health and Social Care and delivers training to national and international practitioners and organisations. He has published in various peer-reviewed areas related to psychotherapy processes and outcomes, trauma and leadership.

Tony McSherry is an existemtial-analytical psychotherapist. His main therapeutic interests are philosophy, existentialism and psychoanalysis. He completed his PhD with Roehampton University, UK.

Peter Meades is a UKCP-registered integrative psychotherapist and IPT-accredited practitioner living in London. He is Head of Counselling/IPT for Cardiff & Vale NHS University Health Board, working remotely supporting a Digital First Service. He has a small private practice in London. As an Hispanophile, he is passionate about the Spanish language, food and culture.

Silva Neves is a COSRT-accredited and UKCP-registered psychosexual and relationship psychotherapist and a trauma psychotherapist. He is a Pink Therapy clinical associate. Silva is Course Director for CICS (Contemporary Institute of Clinical Sexology) and speaks internationally. He is a member of the editorial board for the leading international journal *Sex and Relationship Therapy*. Silva is the author of *Compulsive Sexual Behaviours, A Psycho-Sexual Treatment Guide for Clinicians* (2021).

Sally Parsloe is a psychotherapist in private practice in London. She has worked in a voluntary organisation and in the NHS.

Gillian Proctor is Lecturer in Counselling and Psychotherapy at the University of Leeds, UK. She is also an independent clinical psychologist, offering psychotherapy, supervision and training. Her interests are in politics, ethics and power. She is currently a research fellow, researching authenticity, belonging and inclusion in online teaching and learning. Before moving to academia, she worked in the NHS for 22 years and was passionate about the relationship between inequalities, deprivation and distress and how the power structures within psychiatry often compounded rather than relieve this distress.

Julian-Pascal Saadi is a specialist counselling psychologist working in a London-based Community Mental Health Team (CMHT) within the National Health Services. He is also part-time Academic Lecturer on the Doctorate in Counselling Psychology at Metanoia Institute, UK. Dr Saadi is a member of Pink Therapy and specialises in working with gender, sexual and relationship diverse (GSRD) people. He runs his own private practice where most of his clinical work is with the wider Queer community. Dr Saadi's research interests include working with diverse sexualities and gender identities in the therapeutic space.

James M. Sedgwick is a UKCP-registered psychotherapist and Senior Lecturer in Counselling and Psychotherapy at Newman University, Birmingham, UK.

Introduction—Diversity, inclusion and culture wars: Everything a psychotherapist should need to know about 'intersectional feminist, trans*, critical race/whiteness, migration, (in)equality, queer, disability, post-colonial, decolonial, approaches and studies' but is too afraid to ask?

Del Loewenthal

'Why can't we explore with clients what we used to be able to?'

This was from a supervisee where her client had described successfully instigating sex with a waiter when she called at night for the hotel's room service and the therapist hesitated exploring this with her client/patient for concern she might be seen as against feminism.

For the psychotherapist/psychological therapist it would appear that notions of diversity and inclusion are both increasingly important, and yet increasingly difficult, to be thought about with their clients. Are such difficulties to do with the biases of the person who is the psychotherapist, and/or could it also sometimes be to do with how diversity, inclusion and related terms are constructed?

Overall, the current quest for 'Diversity and Inclusion' might be seen by many as both for the good yet complex. However, for others to question how diversity and inclusion are conceptualised can be unacceptable as it questions their very right to exist, and for yet others to get involved in any culture wars is to fiddle while Rome (the World) burns. Furthermore, this quest for diversity and inclusion can too frequently lead to culture war brick walling.

Crucially, our inability to be clear ourselves on issues of diversity and inclusion as psychotherapists may threaten our very project. This has been where traditionally clients have been able to come to us to explore what they can't elsewhere. For clients may now find it difficult to find a therapist who is able to explore with them their concerns around diversity and inclusion which can be complicated and may take time to consider.

So when is it diversity and when is it perversity and who decides? Similarly, who and what should be included and excluded from what and by whom? Other questions include whether these changes, in what might be considered cultural practices, become permanent or will they, as historically, continue to vary?

Indeed, our liquid modernity (Bauman, 2000) would appear to be bringing increasing instability to both clients and their therapists. To give a further example, there are reports from the consulting room of therapists not daring to question what appears to be a growing number of clients wishing to have a sex change. While hopefully in practice case specific, therapists seem less able to wonder, for example, if the client by changing gender is desperately hoping for a new self, as Kierkegaard (1989 [1849]) describes the wrong reasons for buying a new coat. Or, to give another possibility, a decreasing ability for therapists to potential questioning whether clients recognising the masculine and feminine in themselves is not necessarily the same as having to be bi, etc.? Instead increasingly and unusually we can be lost for words.

How then do we explore our changing world which is so different to the one we were born into (let alone our, often older, own psychotherapists and supervisors)? So are psychotherapists no longer being appropriately curious for fear of being caught in trip wires? Do then psychotherapists need if not a 'trip advisor' somewhere where they can confidentially explore where they are as people and practitioners? The idea of this book which is based on a special issue of the European Journal of Psychotherapy and Counselling (EJPC) in association with the United Kingdom Council of Psychotherapy (UKCP) is that we present research on the cutting edge of these important developments. The intention here is that readers can have the opportunity to explore where they are in themselves and in their therapeutic practices regarding developments in diversity and inclusion.

Regarding the title of this Introduction, it was inspired by an advertisement for a lecturer that asked for the candidate to have expertise in 'intersectional feminist, trans*, critical race/whiteness, migration, (in)equality, queer, disability, post-colonial, decolonial, approaches and studies' (https://www.jobs.ac.uk/job/CQJ949/). The post was in Critical Studies which can be seen as being 'concerned with the ways in which literature and other cultural media reinforce or undermine the economic, political, social, and psychological oppression of people …' (Nickerson, 2022). Yet, as already indicated, are these notions both important and increasingly difficult for psychotherapists (amongst others) to think about with their clients? Furthermore, again as mentioned, are these difficulties both to do with the biases of the person who is the psychotherapist, and could it also sometimes be to do with how these terms are constructed (Loewenthal, 2022; Murray, 2019)?

Before introducing the chapters, I thought it might be helpful to provide at least one definition of these concepts from the title of this Introduction:

Intersectional feminist

A prism for seeing the way in which various forms of inequality often operate together and exacerbate each other.

(Crenshaw, 2023)

Trans

An umbrella term to describe people whose gender is not the same as, or does not sit comfortably with, the sex they were assigned at birth. Trans people may describe themselves using one or more of a wide variety of terms, including (but not limited to) transgender, non-binary, or genderqueer. (stonewall.org.uk)

Whiteness theory

Whiteness theory is a lens used in Whiteness studies that identifies what White identity means in terms of social, political, racial, economic, culture, etc.

(Hartmann et al., 2009)

Critical race theory

Whiteness theory is an offshoot of critical race theory that sees race as a social construct. It posits that practice of Whiteness are visible systems of whiteness that white people use to maintain power to benefit only white people.

(Gabriel, 1998)

See also Kendi (2019) for an emphasis not solely in terms of whiteness. Rather than while race is socially constructed this is according to systems of power rooted in identity which in the West have been constructed to favour certain identities and to prejudice others.

Gender inequality

Men earn more than women, work less, and occupy more of the top jobs – but women live longer, are better educated and get to retire younger. How best to harness the talents of both sexes for better lives all round?

(OECD)

Queer

Queer is an umbrella term for people who are not heterosexual or cisgender. Originally meaning "strange" or "peculiar", queer came to be used pejoratively against those with same-sex desires or relationships in the late 19th century. Beginning in the late 1980s, queer activists, such as the members of Queer

Nation, began to reclaim the word as a deliberately provocative and politically radical alternative to the more assimilationist branches of the LGBT community.

(Sycamore, 2008)

Cisgender

Cisgender (often shortened to cis; sometimes cissexual) is a term used to describe a person whose gender identity corresponds to their sex assigned at birth.

(Merriam-Webster.com Dictionary)

Disability

Persons with disabilities include those with long-term physical, mental, intellectual or sensory impairments which in interaction with various barriers may hinder [a person's] full and effective participation in society on an equal basis with others.

(United Nations Convention on the Rights of Persons with Disabilities)

Postcolonialism

Postcolonialism offers a language of and for those who have no place, who seem not to belong, of those whose knowledges and histories are not allowed to count. It is above all this preoccupation with the oppressed, with the subaltern classes, with minorities in any society, with the concerns of those who live or come from elsewhere, that constitutes the basis of postcolonial politics and remains the core that generates its continuing power.

(Young, 2003)

Decolonial

Decolonial approaches, methods, and movements seek to disrupt colonial and settler-colonial logic and the seeming 'naturalness' of racial capitalism.

(William & Mary)

However, there are many disagreements as to these definitions. For example, with regard to gender inequality there would appear to be an increasing number of people who would want to agree with the statement:

I personally feel that the feminist movement must dream of even more than the elimination of the oppression of women. It must dream of the elimination of obligatory sexualities and sex roles. The dream I find most compelling is one of an androgynous and genderless (though not sexless) society, in which one's sexual anatomy is irrelevant to who one is, what one does, and with whom one makes love.

(Rubin, 1990 [1975])

Yet there are those who are concerned of the detrimental effects of such changes on the development of children and young people. There is also the view developed by James Sedgwick in his chapter for this special issue:

> 'Putatively radical assertions about understanding minority group experience are shown to actually exclude valuable ways of understanding social disadvantage which might better enhance our understanding and efficacy '
> (Sedgwick, 2023)

So it's not that so long as we carry on as we have been trained, for example, encouraging the client to be themselves, that it will all be necessarily alright.

There are also those who see who we are being, for example, regarding gender roles, brought about by our social systems and yet others who think that biological determinism has to be prioritised.

So can we or should we accept as diversity and inclusion those whose views we do not agree with what we think of as acceptable diversity and inclusion? Is there a danger that we get caught in cultural wars where one side sustains and develops inequalities and the other side leads unwanted industrial workers into voting for 'democratic fascism' (Badiou, 2019; Reeves, 2022). Importantly when, as a psychotherapist, is what one's clients raise regarding diversity and inclusion none of our business; when can one just focus on how we've already been trained to work; and, when is it our responsibility to say or even to do something?

To take a final (though difficult) example, there are now legal systems in many countries that can potentially wrongly and rightly influence what might be seen as fundamental to our work as psychotherapists, namely timing and judgement. As psychotherapists, when there might be a concern for safeguarding young and vulnerable adults or preventing the spread of terrorism we can professionally be far better off to report this immediately rather than thoughtfully considering the particular situation. Such forms of discrimination and exclusion can prevent the too many horror stories that do happen; but, can we also at times ruin the lives of our clients and their families by our own lack of abilities to stay with what we haven't worked through ourselves?

It is, for all the above reasons, hoped that readers of this book will have the opportunity to be clearer about the different perspectives of our contributors which may not be their own.

Before finally introducing this book's chapters, I want to acknowledge the following for their invaluable assistance in developing this special issue: Evrinomy Avdi, Gauri Chauhan, Ellen Dunn (and the UKCP Research Group), Anastasios Gaitanidis, Miranda Kersley, Saskia Keville, Anthony McSherry, Elizabeth Nicholl, Gillian Proctor, Francesca Robertson, Daniel Rubenstein, Patricia Talens, Jay Watts, Jean Wells and David Winter. Also, special thanks to our new Assistant Editor William Horsnell.

Next, before concluding and with grateful thanks to the contributors, an introduction to their chapters is as follows:

Our first Chapter is *Queer Minds Queer Needs* by Julian-Pascal Saadi and Erene Hadjiioannou. The authors consider what 'Queering' psychotherapy might mean in order to support the growing number of individuals identifying as LGBTQIA+. They propose that binary thinking restricts understanding these clients' needs and generates insufficient models of care. Instead, they advocate a practice of fluidity, rather than rigidity, to support equitable, anti-oppressive and inclusive practice. As one reviewer commented, 'It feels an important piece of work and well articulated. It will be a great addition to the journal'.

Chapter 2 is *Therapy and Diversity – An (un)therapeutic relationship?* by James Sedwick. This chapter concludes by suggesting that the multiple difficulties within the profession's embrace of diversity can be understood in terms of a refusal to reconsider the theoretical, economic and organisational foundations of our therapeutic work to which questions of diversity pose a serious challenge. A case is made for a more open discussion of the relevant issues with some thoughts given to how revised professional structures might support better practice. As a reviewer comments:

> Thank you for writing this great article. I think you're making the strong point – among several other cutting observations for the complacent (for example, why are some diversity categories passed over?) – that entrenched social and historical realities can't be glossed as being susceptible to change just through "self-awareness" and relational therapeutic work (and those of us who do that are slipping into a kind of solipsistic anaesthetised way of being with others).

Chapter 3 is *A Psychotherapist's Lived Experience In Session with an Asylum Seeker and Translator: An Autoethnographic Case Study* by Nicole Chew-Helbig. Featured in this chapter is a psychotherapy case study recounted from the lived experience of this psychotherapist working with an asylum seeker from Afghanistan, with the help of a translator. The methodology used is an aesthetic inquiry adapted from Autoethnography, which engages the practitioner as the researcher-autoethnographer who enters a 'field', which is the therapy situation.

I would like to quote one of our reviewers at length: 'The auto ethnographic approach adopted by this article is seen as a way of integrating a number of strands and concerns that tend to be left out of the more traditional case study research. By entangling theory and the story while paying attention to the direct experience of the therapist, the article attempts to capture nuances of interaction that are by definition non-verbal and non-communicative. This is a deftly written text that explores a therapeutic encounter that starts from the premise that the client and the therapist do not share a common language.

While in this case, the reasons for this are specific to the biographies of the actors, what is being explored here is the possibility of something happening that cannot be put into words, which nevertheless is crucial for the therapy. By drawing on Gestalt, field theory and the relational approaches to case studies this text presents a tightly argued claim for paying attention to presence rather than representation. The success of this article is in showing that auto ethnography can be a practical methodology, especially in situations where the client's suffering is caused not only by external conditions but also by their experience of being outside of language. This article will be of value to therapists seeking to capture their experience of staying with a client's suffering when this suffering cannot be put into words. It will also be a timely contribution to the emergent field of auto ethnographic case studies'.

Next Chapter 4 is *Being Seen? The lived experience of psychodynamic practitioners disclosing or not disclosing sight impairment* by Laura Evers. Here, the taboo of therapist self-disclosure and literature addressing disclosure and disability issues from a psychodynamic perspective is explored using Interpretative Phenomenological Analysis. Results indicated that an inverse relationship between likelihood to self disclose sight impairment and the extent to which practitioners work with unconscious process and transference. There seems much here we can learn from those with sight impairment about therapy in general. As a reviewer comments, 'Thank you for this research which I found enlightening and interesting to read, and from which I take reflective thoughts about impairment, therapy and self-disclosure'.

Chapter 5 is *How might psychotherapy improve its service to disabled people and people with physical impairment?* by Sally Parsloe. This chapter, which a reviewer describes as an 'Excellent paper', considers how psychotherapy might better serve disabled people and people with physical impairment. It is argued that psychotherapy stands accused of making things worse for people living with physical impairment. Exploration of the articulation by Freud and Lacan of the emergence of subjectivity reveals the reason for the distrust of the disability studies community. However, it is further argued that phenomenology as elucidated by Heidegger and Levinas together with the will to self-critique, offer a way of working that can move to an appropriate respect and service from psychotherapy for disabled people.

The following Chapter 6 is *Towards an Integrative Model of Multicultural Responsiveness* by Daryl Mahon. Here, it is argued that there is an increasing need for practitioners to be responsive to multicultural identities in clinical practice. Yet, the multicultural competency framework, which has been around for a number of decades, overall utility and generalisability have not being consistently established. As a response, both an integrative model of multicultural responsiveness that brings together trans-theoretical practices from the extant literature and a case vignette demonstrating the application and utility of this model are provided. As a reviewer writes, 'This is an important paper; summarising research in the area of cultural competence, critiquing a competency-based model and offering the foundation of an alternative approach which is much needed'.

Chapter 7 is *Deconstructing Humanitarian Compassion* by Artemis Christinaki. This chapter explores humanitarian compassion within the Derridean notion of hospitality. Reflecting on the age of Imperial Humanitarianism where Evangelists formed administrative missions to save the souls of the slaves in the colonial provinces of Europe, it is aimed to address the link of compassion with Christianity and colonialism. Challenging compassion and aid, as they are constituted in psychological discourse, this paper invites therapists to rethink first the contextualisation under which these ideals emerged in the psychological discourse and, second, to introduce a discussion on what psychology does to refugees as well as 'counselling minorities'. As a reviewer comments, 'This is an excellent paper that should be published … the paper is interesting, thoughtful, clear and well written'.

Next Chapter 8 is *Diversity and aggression: a reflection on sensual meanings and an ameliorative law after Freud and Lacan* by Tony McSherry. The aim of this chapter is to explore phenomenologically how the 'inside' (psychical) and 'outside' (the other and/or society) interweave following the concern that sometimes those of us who favour diversity may also inadvertently shut it down. The concern is raised that if we cannot hear our own thoughts that come to us from the 'inside', then how can we move towards diversity on the 'outside'. Two fictional accounts are given from everyday life. A reviewer commented, 'I loved this article, thought it was very moving, well written with beautiful (phenomenological) description of difference and addressing the aggression in all of us, signifying the need for space for thoughtfulness'.

Chapter 9, the last chapter before introducing the chapters of our published respondents, is *An Exploration of Lesbian and Gay People's Experiences of Religion, and their Implications for Psychotherapy: An Interpretative Phenomenological Analysis* by Peter Meades.

This research, which a reviewer considers, 'A great paper and very well written', explores lesbian and gay people's experiences of Christianity, Islam and Judaism and the implications for psychotherapy in the context of a wider social discourse regarding heterosexist hegemony. This project is considered to have the potential to increase psychotherapists' awareness of the intersection of homosexuality and religion and the diverse ways in which this plays out. Here, therapists are invited to consider any potentially socially constructed positions and encourage a life-course perspective.

Chapter 10, from our first published respondent Silva Neves, is entitled *Contemporary psychotherapy: evolution in our modern time – A response.* Silva argues that change and learning are necessary to keep a contemporary psychotherapy practice; however, change is difficult because allowing ourselves to face our 'blind spots' may provoke shame. Thus, it is important for psychotherapists to be robust and manage the discomfort of learning. It is with this frame of mind that Silva comments on the previous chapters. A reviewer commented, 'Overall I thought that this was a brilliant introduction to this edition of the journal. I thought that it nicely sets up … various points of inquiry that are explored in more detail … '.

Chapter 11, our second published response, is *Diversity in Counselling and Psychotherapy* by Gillian Proctor. Here, on commentating on the chapters, Gillian critiques the concepts of 'diversity' and 'inclusion' promoting a critical diversity approach. Gillian further raises the concept of 'ableism' as an issue with a plea for ongoing deconstruction of language and attention to inequalities both within and without the profession. As a reviewer comments, 'In this powerful and thought-provoking commentary … the author argues for a critical diversity approach and critiques the way in which diversity and inclusion concepts are sometimes used'.

Complex topics, such as diversity and inclusion, cannot often be dealt with quickly, and we very much hope this book will provide much needed information for us as psychological therapists to put our clients first. As Editor-in-Chief of the EJPC I explored a similar topic 'Enabling Difference' (Loewenthal, 2003). That was almost 20 years ago, and while this might now be seen as pioneering, there was not then as currently either such evidence of culture wars or being lost for words. It is very much hoped that the chapters here will aid helping us as psychotherapists to find the words for ourselves and our clients so we can better know when we are being inappropriately, and when we are being appropriately, curious and when we are too scared to be, but should be, curious regarding issues of diversity and inclusion.

References

Badiou, A. (2019). *Trump*. Polity Press.

Bauman, Z. (2000). *Liquid modernity*. Blackwell.

Crenshaw, K. W. (2023). *On intersectionality: Essential writings*. The New Press.

Gabriel, J. (1998). *Whitewash: Racialized politics and the media*. Routledge.

Hartmann, D., Gerteis, J., & Croll, P. R. (2009). An empirical assessment of whiteness theory: Hidden from how many? *Social Problems*, 56(3), 403–424. https://doi.org/10.1525/sp.2009.56.3.403

jobs.ac.uk. Retrieved June 8, 2022, from https://www.jobs.ac.uk/job/CQJ949/lecturer-in-social-sciences-interdisciplinary-studies-full-time-36-months-fixed-term?uuid=288be114-e6cd-11ec-a349-064da8edb92a&campaign=jbe20220608&source=jbe

Kendi, I. X. (2019). *How to be an antiracist*. One World.

Kierkegaard, S. (19891849). *The sickness unto death*. (A. Hannay, Trans.). Penguin.

Loewenthal, D. (2003). Jacques Derrida and enabling difference: 'Let's talk turkey' [editorial]. *European Journal of Psychotherapy, Counselling and Health*, 6(4), 265–267. https://doi.org/10.1080/13642530412331325011

Loewenthal, D. (2022). Psychotherapy and healthy masculinity: Exploring our values, and what stops us thinking about them, when working psychotherapeutically with increasingly unstable notions of masculinity. *European Journal of Psychotherapy & Counselling*, 24(2), 155–161. https://doi.org/10.1080/13642537.2022.2089961

Merriam-Webster. Retrieved October 29, 2022, from https://www.merriam-webster.com/dictionary/cisgender

Murray, D. (2019). *The madness of crowds: Gender, race and identity*. Bloomsbury.

Nickerson, C. (2022, January 6). Understanding critical theory. *Simply Psychology*. www.simplypsychology.org/critical-theory.html

OECD. Retrieved October 29, 2022, from https://www.oecd.org/development/genderinequality.htm

Reeves, R. (2022). *Of boys and men: Why the modern male is struggling, why it matters, and what to do about it*. (Great Britain) Swift Press.

Rubin, G. (19901975). The traffic in women: Notes on the "political economy" of sex. In K. Hansen & I. Philipson (Eds.), *Women, class, and the feminist imagination* (pp. 74–113). Temple.

Sedgwick, J. (2023). Therapy and diversity – an (un)therapeutic relationship? *European Journal of Psychotherapy and Counselling*. 25:1–2, 29–43, DOI: 10.1080/13642537.2022.2156158

stonewall.org.uk. Retrieved October 29, 2022, from https://www.stonewall.org.uk/what-does-trans-mean

Sycamore, M. (2008). *That's revolting!: Queer strategies for resisting assimilation*. Soft Skull Press.

United Nations. https://www.un.org/development/desa/disabilities/convention-on-the-rights-of-persons-with-disabilities/article-1-purpose.html

William & Mary. Retrieved October 29, 2022, from https://www.wm.edu/sites/dhp/decoloniality/index.php

Young, R. (2003). *Postcolonialism: A very short introduction*. Oxford University Press.

Queer minds, Queer needs

Erene Hadjiioannou and Julian-Pascal Saadi

ABSTRACT

Equal access to mental healthcare is a right held by all Britons, yet evidence suggests that individuals from the LGBTQIA + population have poorer experiences compared to cisgender and heterosexual clients. This is problematic when considered alongside the impact of living in a societally disempowering world. Research highlights how our mental health systems perpetuate harm to LGBTQIA+ patients. One of these systems is the institution and practice of psychotherapy. We draw on our three fold positionalities to explore what change in the practice of psychotherapy could look like. Specifically, we consider what 'Queering' psychotherapy might mean in order to support the growing number of individuals identifying as LGBTQIA+. We also reflect on the binaries underpinning our discipline and discuss their role in perpetuating harm during psychotherapy. We propose that binary thinking restricts understanding our clients' needs and generates insufficient models of care. We advocate a practice of fluidity, rather than rigidity, to support equitable practice. By 'Queering' psychotherapy provision in Britain, we contribute to the evidence base for anti-oppressive and inclusive practice.

Introduction

It is established that Queer people have greater mental health needs compared to cisgender and heterosexual people (Chakraborty et al., 2011; Dhejne et al., 2016; Sandfort et al., 2001). Evidence also suggests that lesbian, gay, and bisexual clients have poorer psychotherapeutic outcomes compared to heterosexual clients (Beard et al., 2017; Plöderl et al., 2017; Rimes et al., 2019), within UK-based public health settings, highlighting a need to reconsider how we provide psychotherapy to Queer clients.

The confidentiality of therapy assumes a space in which clients speak freely, relatively uninhibited by fear, shame, and guilt (Younggren & Harris,

2008). However, this space is one amongst many we occupy as members of a binarised society. These binaries restrict our understanding of ourselves and others (Iantaffi & Barker, 2019). In psychotherapy, binaries can create barriers for Queer clients, manifesting as difficulties in accessibility and engagement. From this we advocate a practice of fluidity, rather than fixed binaries.

By 'Queer', we use a western, affirmative umbrella term to refer to people who fall outside the categories of cisgender, heterosexual, and/or monogamous. This widens the scope of a commonly-used term, LGBT (lesbian, gay, bisexual, transgender), denoting the diverse ways people experience their gender, sexuality, and relationship style. The ways in which these are expressed are, we believe, forms of subverting or refusing oppressive societal norms and reclaiming power. This paper focuses on gender and sexuality, but its principles can be extended to supporting work with fluidity and diversity in relationship styles.

Positionality

We as authors hold a threefold position: we are Queer, currently work with Queer-identified clients, and have accessed mental health services ourselves as Queer people. Julian-Pascal identifies as a mixed-heritage, White-presenting, middle class, cisgender man. Erene identifies as a cisgender, middle class, Greek Cypriot, White woman.

We recognise the ease of publicly identifying as cisgender and White (normative and visible identities, respectively) including how they protect and accommodate us within many spaces. We often sit or are placed on one side of a gender and race binary, but the same cannot be said about our queerness.

We know the potential negative impact of publicly outing the specifics of our queerness in a binary society. Here we use silence as a 'resource [used by] Queer people ... to survive' (Hammoud-Beckett, 2007, p. 36). Instead of being silenced, we choose to be silent on the specifics of our queerness here.

Positioning ourselves acknowledges that our identities contextualise lived experiences, which in turn enter professional spaces, including writing this article. We encourage readers to assess their positionalities also.

Social context

Matters specific to the Queer community are debated and polarised on a public scale in the United Kingdom. As distressed Queer clients are forced to engage with intersections of policy, law, and health care, so are we as psychotherapists trying to meet their needs. In this section, we summarise the societal and psychotherapeutic legacy of pathologising queerness.

The medical model of psychological distress around gender moved diagnostic criteria from transsexualism to gender dysphoria (American Psychiatric Association, 2013). Homosexuality was removed from the Diagnostic and Statistical Manual of Mental Disorders in 1974. Public opposition against conversion therapy in the U.K. is the latest version of social justice challenging harmful practices that deny gender variance (Haldeman, 2022).

Despite these changes, gender and sexuality largely continue to be medically organised by the male/female and straight/gay binaries, for example: only making reference to experiencing oneself as 'the other' gender (American Psychiatric Association, 2013), which can pose problems to the Queer community.These pathologising legacies shape how psychotherapists respond to Queer clients and the extent to which they can hope to be supported.

As an alternative, conceptualising gender and sexuality as psychobiosocial is one way that the binary has been destabilised. For example, Richards and Barker (2013) suggest that gender combines internal experiences of one's identity, biological factors (such as: genetics, hormones, chromosomes, gonads, and anatomy), as well as normative values espoused by society on what gender 'should' be.

Mainstream services are not typically set up to think about the complexity of 'queerness', meaning that Queer clients often seek LGBT+ specific services as a substitute (Bachman & Gooch, 2018). Within the National Health Service (NHS), for example, referral pathways for therapy are typically informed by diagnosis and interventions are delivered accordingly. This follows the scientific evidence-base outlined by the National Institute for Health and Care Excellence.

Although there are therapies which promote the kind of values (i.e. non-pathologising, non-judgemental) discussed in this paper (e.g. person centred or existential therapy, feminist therapy, or interventions centering racialised trauma), they are not often available in the NHS. Clauses within ethical codes of conduct similarly emphasise non-discrimination of protected characteristics, but in practice 'queerness' often falls through the gaps of systemic inconsistencies in care.

However, there are increasing numbers of medical and allied health professionals who include social context, power, and intersectionality into their treatment plans. An example of this is the demand for cultural competence trainings, and the use of the Power Threat Meaning Framework in trauma-informed services (Johnston & Boyle, 2018).

Under the medical model, societal and relational oppressions experienced in response to ones' identity do not always enter the psychotherapeutic space. This can be problematic if symptoms of psychological distress are the result of not being able to consistently live in one's identity without negative consequences. From this, a binary within psychotherapy emerges, one that decouples the internal (psychological) from the external (social) world pointing to a need for integration.

To offset this, psychotherapy could adopt a fluid stance that challenges binary systems and practices in a way that meets the needs that some Queer clients present with (Moon, 2010). For readers that do not already, we encourage reflecting on the following question: How will you bring sexual and gender identity into the therapeutic space?

Formation of Queer minds and the binary

Identity formation is created within a dynamic interpersonal process throughout one's lifetime (Page & Peacock, 2013). Positive value is emphasised for non-Queer identities in society meaning Queer people often navigate becoming themselves in privacy (at least initially), lacking affirming social narratives and role modelling around queerness (Fraser, 2009; Lev, 2009).

In this context, it is up to Queer people to seek mentors and guidance, and engage in activism to meet their needs. Examples include: Queer bookshops, online forums, Queer zines and blogs, anti-oppressive therapist networks, and YouTube videos. These double as a safe haven promoting growth, affirmation, and validation.

Alarmingly, some communities' resources (e.g. trans-specific forums) have been weaponised by some to construe that online forums are causing a social contagion of transness among young persons. This has been used to explain a 'sudden' rise in referrals to gender identity clinics, a phenomenon framed as 'rapid-onset gender dysphoria' (ROGD) (Ashley, 2020). Proponents of ROGD theory suggest that support forums induce false beliefs into the minds of distressed young persons, causing them to believe that transitioning will provide a concrete solution to their distress. For them, a young person coming out as transgender is evidence that they are not transgender: they are merely misplacing distress.

The above example illustrates the vicious cycle created by cis-heteronormativity. That is, in oppressing Queer people these systems create a need for community-based resources to survive. However, this becomes pathologised by those unwilling to think about the influence of cis-heteronormativity in shaping their perception of reality. An insidious loop thus creates itself, culminating in pathologising of the basic human need for connection with 'similar others'.

The lack of consistently affirmative social narratives around Queer identity is based on cis-heteronormativity, creating a world organised by straightness and the male/female dichotomy. If one identifies outside of these norms (e.g. bisexual or transgender), one risks being assigned negative stereotypes associated with sexual and gender variance. Therefore, binaries are partly responsible for the distress Queer clients present with since they perpetuate discrimination.

The issue of binaries in psychotherapy has been explored and deconstructed elsewhere (e.g. Moon, 2010). However, an important idea to reiterate is that: if 'normality' is defined under a binary, then Queer identity necessarily develops in conflict with normality (Fraser, 2009). Feelings of alienation and social isolation are common among Queer youth, and one reason for this may be a lack of similar others accessible to the same degree as cisgender, heterosexual, and/or monogamous people. Although social media has started to change this for those that have access to it, Burns (2018) reminds us of the pre-internet age during which many relied on word of mouth and letters in the post to connect with other Queer people. Additionally, many people globally have limited access to social media, the internet, or devices that connect to the internet.

Fraser (2009) describes how the unseen self develops, relates, connects, and trusts in relation to transgender youth. They suggest that a 'faulty mirroring happens during periods of identity construction because the transgender self is often invisible to the outside world' (p. 126). When Queer children do not have parents who mirror same-sex or gender diverse feelings, a 'false self' is affirmed instead. This can make it more difficult for some Queer youth to know what queerness is and how they want to live it. Although referring to a time where access to digital platforms or LGBTQIA+ societies in schools was limited, Fraser's ideas still arguably apply to digitally excluded groups or less inclusive schools.

Early experiences of inadequate mirroring combined with ventures into a society with fixed lines between acceptable/not acceptable can create internalised homophobia, transphobia, lesbophobia, biphobia, etc (Sue, 2010). Considering the impact of internalised oppression on our clients' mental health can be validating and important within therapy.

The intersections of religion, ethnicity and culture can exacerbate pressures of binary thinking. Das Nair (2008) reference Black and ethnic-minority Queer identities as an example of the challenges created at such intersections within the U.K. High rates of conversion practices in religious communities demonstrates another harm this intersection can create (Haldeman, 2022). Finally, patriarchal sexism compounds notions of cisgender as normative and men as dominant, potentially explaining why transgender women (rather than transgender men) are aggressively targeted by the media and radical feminist groups (Faye, 2021).

The implications of 'straightness' and 'cisness'

Understanding society's binary underpinnings of sexuality and gender requires thinking about 'straightness' and 'cisness'. Richards and Barker (2013) note that cisgender people have little opportunity to reflect on their gender because it develops in line with cisnormative affirmations. Assuming that cisness is normal becomes ingrained and automatically upheld, similar to heterosexuality and their limited opportunities to consider 'straightness'.

Typical narratives around gender include men struggling to express emotions and not asking for help, or women struggling to put themselves first (Richards & Barker, 2013). Adherence to the gender binary thus shapes one's way of being in the world, even if this causes psychological distress. For example, men have higher rates of completed suicides which has been linked to difficulties with help-seeking and emotional expression (Möller-Leimkühler, 2003).

In psychotherapy we may solely assess clients' difficulties in expressing and regulating emotions from a developmental lens, demonstrating inadequate examination of cisness and straightness. Not considering gender role socialisation can thus limit understanding our clients. Readers may consider times when cisgender and heterosexual clients felt the pressure to conform to traditional milestones of marriage and having children, for example, even when this was not their desire.

Although reflective practice is a core component of psychotherapeutic work, this rarely extends to discussing straightness or cisness. Overlooking these concepts within psychotherapy trainings and health services forces the Queer community to step up once more to educate and create change.

Working example: Genders beyond the binary

For the purpose of this article, we use the term 'transgender' to refer to people whose gender identity is different to that which they were assigned at birth. In the U.K this is based on the male/female binary, determined by the appearance of external genitalia. Whilst psychotherapists arguably deal with minds rather than bodies, the way we gender bodies at birth reinforces a societal binary informed by rigid cisnormative values. In this section, 'transgender' may include: transgender men, women, and non-binary people; a-gender, bi-gender, and fluidly gendered people – and beyond (Richards & Barker, 2013).

Evidence suggests that clients from the transgender community are some of the most neglected among Queer folk when accessing healthcare (Rees et al., 2020). Genders outside of the binary may be pathologised when unexamined, resulting in othering and creating an atmosphere of mistrust which then poses barriers to accessibility. It raises the question of what a health service could look like if we committed to rethinking our understanding of 'healthy'. As poignantly asked by Sharman (2021, p. 12):

> What if all health care providers and healers genuinely honoured and valued queer and trans people, worked collaboratively with us, and trusted in our expert knowledge of our own bodies? ... What if the care we received was rooted in a commitment to our liberation and the liberation of all people?

An example of the influence of cis-normativity transpires in the framing of transness as a symptom of trauma or underlying difficulties (e.g. Evans & Evans, 2021). An inductive leap posits a need for 'treatment' to restore the 'true' cisgender identity, denying the possibility that gender variance is healthy and in turn exposing cis-normativity as an organising structure. This pathologising approach echoes the problems faced by the homosexual community in the 20th century, recently being considered a type of conversion therapy by the U.K. government (Government Equalities Office & Equality Hub, 2021).

We hold a nuanced view, recognising that trauma often forces reconfiguration of the self, which can be a normal response to experiences such as abuse (Hadjiioannou, 2021). A change in one's sense of self, including gender identity, after trauma does not necessarily equate to a 'symptom' that must be alleviated. Rather, it is a change in one's relationship to their identity which is worth exploring as part of processing the impact of traumatic experiences in therapy.

Diagnostic criteria for gender dysphoria (American Psychiatric Association, 2013) acknowledge that a person's desires and behaviours may be of an alternative gender to the one assigned at birth, but there remains a focus on 'the other' gender, reinforcing the male/female binary rather than a gender spectrum. As a medical intervention, diagnosis is followed by hormones and/or surgery. Whilst these interventions often alleviate distress, and barriers to treatment can exacerbate distress (World Professional Association for Transgender Health, 2012), unexplored adherence to this binary reinforces homogenisation of what 'transgender' means. It reinforces fixed ideas that: 1) transgender is a mental health issue requiring treatment, and 2) treatment needs to involve changing one's body. The pathologising legacy of the transsexual model is thus upheld despite an evolved diagnosis (Coolhart et al., 2008).

We have had conversations with multiple transgender clients about how this community is tasked with building the health system it needs, often trying to pass within the male/female binary to do so due to hegemonic gender roles (Richards et al., 2018). This has been weaponised by some to assert that trans people maintain the binary in their adherence to sexist stereotypes (Greer, 1999; Hausman, 1995). This unhelpfully allocates blame to another oppressed group, thus maintaining the system partly responsible for such stereotypes in the first place (cis-heteronormativity).

Even if gaining a gender dysphoria diagnosis is reassuring, the process is rarely risk-free to transgender clients who already live in a binary world that is not risk-free. The safety of the psychotherapeutic space becomes delicate and easily negated. We must do better to manage distress produced by tensions between fluid Queer inner realities and outer binary realities.

Psychotherapy as a fluid system

Many regulatory guidelines for psychotherapy state the importance of being non-judgemental to ethically support all clients. Within a binary society, however, we adhere to fixed ideas on: how we understand clients, how clients should engage with services, and what successful treatment looks like. In doing so we risk overlooking sub-sections of Queer clients who bypass the binary entirely, such as: asexual, intersex, and bisexual people.

Adhering to a non-judgemental stance arguably includes unlearning binary principles which permeate our sense of self/other and regulate our behaviour when thought about as systems of power. Binary thinking misleads us to privilege one identity over the other (e.g. heterosexual over homosexual), which shapes and informs how we 'do' psychotherapy (Zeeman et al., 2014). Clients could cease to be categorised as well/unwell, heterosexual/homosexual, or male/female, instead being offered space to flexibly express who they are. It can be important to adopt this stance with Queer clients because binaries can impact the quality of healthcare experiences (Rees et al., 2020; Sharman, 2021).

Barriers to accessing Queer-affirmative psychotherapy are dictated by finances. If a Queer person can afford private psychotherapy they can pick a professional who is explicitly Queer-affirmative for support. This is not so for those with less financial privilege, and for whom finding queer-affirmative psychotherapy is down to what is locally available.

Queer identities rarely fit rigid, binary categories, indicating a need for flexible understandings of 'queerness' (Moon, 2010). Binaries also risk homogenising sub-sections of the Queer community, for example transgender being misconstrued as only ever indiciating male-to-female or female-to-male. Without therapeutic spaces enabling exploration of gender diverse feelings, a Queer client may succumb to the oppressive binary illusion that only two types of trans 'becoming' exist. Occupying a fluid psychotherapeutic stance might include seeking, welcoming, and incorporating input from transgender communities to meet the full range of trans needs. This extends the spirit of allyship to increase accessibility and empowerment.

There is also a growing amount of evidence challenging the straight/gay binary. Terms such as 'straight-ish and 'mostly straight' highlight that categories of 'straightness' are being challenged (Savin-Williams, 2017). Millenials are also less likely to define themselves within with the straight/gay binary because these categories have pathologising legacies that fail to capture their lived experiences.

From this, psychotherapists learn that traditional descriptors such as 'transgender', 'cisgender, 'gay', or 'straight' cannot necessarily be taken at face value. Empowering all clients to self-define allows for exploration of the specific meanings of categories they choose. This supports clients to foster connections between the different aspects of their sense of self. It also assists the psychotherapist in having a clearer understanding of who their client is and what they need from them.

Implications for clinical practice

If, as a member of a society organised by binary systems, a psychotherapist brings limited understandings of gender and sexuality into the room the implications are multiple.

Primarily, the assumed protective boundary of confidentiality creates a vacuum in which psychological harm may occur when psychotherapists do not trouble the systems of cis-heteronormativity. The result is a repetition of developmental and societal impingements in which internal reality is not affirmed by the external world (Fraser, 2009). This can compromise the reparative nature of psychotherapeutic contact if it generates feelings of unsafety, rejection, or hypervigilance. Furthermore, many therapists do not support the banning of conversion therapy for transgender people further reinforcing the idea that safety is not always guaranteed.

Richards and Barker (2013) recognise that Queer clients seek psychotherapy for different reasons. Sometimes their presenting concerns are explicitly linked to their gender/sexual/relationship identities, and at other times are irrelevant. Establishing this at the outset avoids making assumptions about what Queer clients need, including avoiding the pathologising assumption that the cause of their concerns are their non-normative identities.

It is our view that: regardless of any explicit request by Queer clients to think about their identity amongst their mental health needs, adopting a minority-stress model (Meyer, 2003) assists in understanding how living in a cis-heteronormative world can erode personal power and expression, as well as comfortable contact with self and other.

Psychotherapeutically, we may discover Queer distress in the form of depression, suicidality, and substance misuse (Bachman & Gooch, 2018). When this occurs, we acknowledge that societal living means exposure to non-affirmative contact, including physical violence (Bachman & Gooch, 2017), which is bound to cause difficulties with living.

Importantly, identity concealment can prevent Queer clients from considering a link between their 'presenting problems' and the impact of living in a cis-heteronormative world. It can thus be helpful to actively bring in sexual orientation/gender identity into the room so as to provide the client with an opportunity to consider the impact of oppression on their mental health, in turn externalising the problem and exposing the toxicity of internalised oppression which can damage self-esteem. This opportunity can always be declined by the client so that the remit of the work remains within their consent.

It is important not to discredit clients who do not link cis-heteronormativity to their difficulties. However, the lack of a link is not always evidence that there is no link. Some links are difficult to make because of the pain they produce, rather than because they do not exist. Confronting the trauma produced by living in an oppressive world is a painful task, but arguably key if we are to support clients to develop more positive relationships with their queerness.

Sensitive, empathic interest about queerness is not centring queerness as part of the problem, as this would reinforce pathologisation. We instead draw the reader's attention to the fact of Queer oppression and the role this has in producing distress. Enquiries about the impact of living in an oppressive world means resisting oppression. This fits with a social justice perspective aiming to empower clients to think about and push back against systemic oppression where safely possible, on their own terms. This may lie in their own private expressions of gender/sexuality, including 'coming out' or 'inviting others in' as a first step (Beckett, 2014; Langridge, 2008).

A final implication is concerned with the impact of cis-heteronormativity on therapists' understanding of Queer distress. All therapists (Queer and non-Queer) are arguably tasked with having to 'Queer' their practice and, by extension, their realities in order to observe the ways in which cis-heteronormativity influences clinical thinking. For example: deconstructing understandings of sexuality/gender, and then seeking to educate themselves by engaging with key Queer authors (e.g. Itantaffi, 2021; Moon, 2008, 2010). This extends a practice of simply having 'add-ons' of knowledge (e.g. one-off trainings or having a 'special interest' in Queer issues), proposing instead a fundamental need to rethink how we 'do' psychotherapy with Queer clients.

As practical steps to Queer one's practice, we suggest mirroring the fluidity of Queer realities by signalling safety, affirmation, and respect throughout therapy. These are some options: asking during assessments what it has been like to access support to contextualise experiences of disempowerment and oppression; adding Queer signifiers (rainbow/progress pride flag); and working together with local Queer communities to co-produce 'culturally competent' interventions. This can include co-delivery with members of the community, so that information and power isn't withheld.

Conclusion

Binary systems of organising gender and sexuality historically oppress Queer clients. Psychotherapists are in excellent positions to offset the disempowering impact of such binaries by adopting more fluid understandings of gender/sexuality. We advocate for psychotherapists to provide Queer clients with a mirror, hearing their story and reflecting it back in order to practise allyship. This can help to humanise and contextualise mental health difficulties, encouraging reparative contact throughout their therapeutic journey.

Disclosure statement

No potential conflict of interest was reported by the authors.

ORCID

Erene Hadjiioannou http://orcid.org/0000-0002-9642-9885

References

American Psychiatric Association. (2013). *Diagnostic and statistical manual of mental disorders* (5th ed.).

Ashley, F. (2020). A critical commentary on 'rapid-onset gender dysphoria'. *The Sociological Review Monographs*, *68*(4), 779–799. https://doi.org/10.1177/0038026120934693

Bachman, C. L., & Gooch, B. (2017). *LGBT in Britain: Hate crime and discrimination*. Stonewall.

Bachman, C. L., & Gooch, B. (2018). *LGBT in Britain: Health report*. Stonewall.

Beard, C., Kirakosian, N., Silverman, A. L., Winer, J. P., Wadsworth, L. P., & Björgvinsson, T. (2017). Comparing treatment response between LGBQ and heterosexual individuals attending a CBT- and DBT-skills-based partial hospital. *Journal of Consulting and Clinical Psychology*, *85*(12), 1171–1181. https://doi.org/10.1037/ccp0000251

Beckett, S. (2014). Azima ila Hayati – An invitation in to my life: Narrative conversations and sexual identity. In M. Lindsay (Ed.), *Counselling ideologies: Queer challenges to heteronormativity* (pp. 201–217). Ashgate Publishing Ltd.

Burns, C. (2018). *Trans Britain: Our journey from the shadows*. Unbound.

Chakraborty, A., McManus, S., Brugha, T. S., Bebbington, P., & King, M. (2011). Mental health of the non-heterosexual population of England. *British Journal of Psychiatry*, *198*(2), 143–148. https://doi.org/10.1192/bjp.bp.110.082271

Coolhart, D., Provancher, N., Hager, A., & Wang, M.-N. (2008). Recommending transsexual clients for gender transition: A therapeutic tool for assessing readiness. *Journal of GLBT Family Studies*, *4*(3), 301–324. https://doi.org/10.1080/15504280802177466

Dhejne, C., Vlerken, R. V., Heylens, G., & Arcelus, J. (2016). Mental health and gender dysphoria: A review of the literature. *International Review of Psychiatry*, *28*(1), 44–57. https://doi.org/10.3109/09540261.2015.1115753

Evans, S., & Evans, M. (2021). *Gender dysphoria: A therapeutic model for working with children, adolescents and young adults*. Phoenix Publishing House Ltd.

Faye, S. (2021). *The transgender issues: An argument for justice*. Penguin Books.

Fraser, L. (2009). Depth psychotherapy with transgender people. *Sexual and Relationship Therapy*, *24*(2), 126–142. https://doi.org/10.1080/14681990903003878

Government Equalities Office & Equality Hub. (2021). *Conversion therapy: An evidence assessment and qualitative study*. https://www.gov.uk/government/publications/conversion-therapy-an-evidence-assessment-and-qualitative-study

Greer, G. (1999). *The whole woman*. Doubleday.

Hadjiioannou, E. (2021). *Psychotherapy with survivors of sexual violence: Inside and outside the room*. Routledge.

Haldeman, D. C. (2022). *The case against conversion "therapy": Evidence, ethics, and alternatives*. American Psychological Association.

Hammoud-Beckett, S. (2007). Azima ila Hayati - An invitation in to my life: Narrative conversations about sexual identity. *The International Journal of Narrative and Community Work*, *1*, 29–39.

Hausman, B. (1995). *Changing sex: Transsexualism, technology, and the idea of gender*. Duke University Press.

Iantaffi, A., & Barker, M. J. (2019). *Life isn't binary: On being both, beyond and in-between*. Jessie Kingsley Publishers.

Itantaffi, A. (2021). *Gender trauma: Healing cultural, social and historical gendered trauma*. Jessica Kingsley Publishers.

Johnston, L., & Boyle, M. (2018). *The power threat meaning framework: Towards the identification of patterns in emotional distress, unusual experiences and troubled or troubling behaviour, as an alternative to functional psychiatric diagnosis*. British Psychological Society.

Langridge, D. (2008). Are you angry or are you heterosexual? A Queer critique of lesbian and gay models of identity development. In L. Moon (Ed.), *Feeling Queer or Queer feelings? Radical approaches to counselling sex, sexualities and genders* (pp. 23–35). Routledge.

Lev, A. I. (2009). *Transgender emergence: Therapeutic guidelines for working with gender-variant people and their families*. Routledge.

Meyer, I. H. (2003). Prejudice, social stress, and mental health in lesbian, gay, and bisexual populations: Conceptual issues and research evidence. *Psychology Bulletin*, *129*(5), 674–697. https://doi.org/10.1037/0033-2909.129.5.674

Möller-Leimkühler, A. M. (2003). The gender gap in suicide and premature death or: Why are men so vulnerable? *European Archives of Psychiatry and Clinical Neuroscience*, *253*(1), 1–8. https://doi.org/10.1007/s00406-003-0397-6

Moon, L. (2008). *Feeling Queer or Queer feelings? Radical approaches to counselling sex, sexualities and genders*. Routledge.

Moon, L. (2010). *Counselling ideologies: Queer challenges to heteronormativity*. Ashgate Publishing Limited.

Nair, R. D. (2008). *Coming out, Staying in, and Stepping in and out of the Closet: Questions of Black and Minority Ethnic-Queer Identities*.

Page, A. D., & Peacock, J. R. (2013). Negotiating identities in a heteronormativecontext. *Journal of Homosexuality*, *60*(4), 639–654. https://doi.org/10.1080/00918369.2012.724632

Plöderl, M., Kunrath, S., Cramer, R. J., Wang, J., Hauer, L., & Fartacek, C. (2017). Sexual orientation differences in treatment expectation, alliance, and outcome among patients at risk for suicide in a public psychiatric hospital. *BMC Psychiatry*, *17*(1), 184–197. https://doi.org/10.1186/s12888-017-1337-8

Rees, S. N., Crowe, M., & Harris, S. (2020). The lesbian, gay, bisexual and transgender communities' mental health care needs and experiences of mental health services: An integrative review of qualitative studies. *Journal of Psychiatric and Mental Health Nursing*, *28*(4), 578–589. https://doi.org/10.1111/jpm.12720

Richards, C., & Barker, M. (2013). *Sexuality and gender for counsellors, psychologists and other health professionals: A practical guide*. Sage.

Richards, C., Barker, M.-J., & Bouman, W. P. (2018). *Genderqueer and non-binary genders: Critical and applied approaches in sexuality, gender and identity*. Palgrave Macmillan.

Rimes, K. A., Ion, D., Wingrove, J., & Carter, B. (2019). Sexual orientation differences in psychological treatment outcomes for depression and anxiety: National cohort study. *Journal of Consulting and Clinical Psychology*, *87*(7), 577–589. https://doi.org/10.1037/ccp0000416

Sandfort, T. G., de Graaf, R., Bijl, R. V., & Schnabel, P. (2001). Same-sex sexual behaviour and psychiatric disorders: Findings from the Netherlands Mental Health Survey and Incidence Study (NEMESIS). *Archives of General Psychiatry*, *58*(1), 85–91. https://doi.org/10.1001/archpsyc.58.1.85

Savin-Williams, R. C. (2017). *Mostly straight: Sexual fluidity among men*. Harvard University Press.

Sharman, Z. (2021). *The care we dream of: Liberatory and transformative approaches to LGBTQ+ health*. Arsenal Pulp Press.

Sue, D. W. (2010). *Microaggressions in everyday life: Race, gender, and sexual orientation*. John Wiley & Sons.

World Professional Association for Transgender Health. (2012). *Standards of care for the health of transsexual, transgender, and gender nonconforming people* (Version 7). https://www.wpath.org/publications/soc

Younggren, J. N., & Harris, E. A. (2008). Can you keep a secret? Confidentiality in psychotherapy. *Journal of Clinical Psychology: In Session, 64*(5), 589–600. https://doi.org/10.1002/jclp.20480

Zeeman, L., Aranda, K., & Grant, A. (2014). *Queering health: Critical challenges to normative health and healthcare.* PCCS Books.

OPEN ACCESS

Therapy and diversity – an (un)therapeutic relationship?

James M. Sedgwick

ABSTRACT

There is fundamental confusion and notable omissions within counselling and psychotherapy's adoption of diversity principles. This prevents the profession from achieving its aims of more respectful and efficacious clinical practice with certain populations. The article argues that uncritical over-reliance on ideas from outside the profession has resulted in a failure to appraise which groups might require specific attention. Unacknowledged confusion between celebratory and critical approaches to diversity is also identified as a source of practical muddle. Putatively radical assertions about understanding minority group experience are shown to actually exclude valuable ways of understanding social disadvantage, which might better enhance our understanding and efficacy. The article concludes by suggesting that the multiple difficulties within the profession's embrace of diversity can be understood in terms of a refusal to reconsider the theoretical, economic and organisational foundations of our therapeutic work to which questions of diversity pose a serious challenge. A case is made for a more open discussion of the relevant issues accompanied by a call for revised professional organization to support knowledge production.

Introduction

The counselling and psychotherapy profession's enthusiasm for discussing issues of diversity proceeds unchecked (with odd, notable exceptions; see Dalal, 2008). Each year brings a fresh crop of publications and workshops, which are warmly endorsed. If consensus was synonymous with correctness, then offering a critical evaluation would be gratuitous.

Our clinical work can only be strengthened by a greater awareness of external circumstances and typical group experience. Unfortunately, the therapy[1] profession perpetually comes up with problematic answers to the right questions when it comes to diversity. Discussions typically perform a regrettable double manoeuvre of both impairing our usual ability to view our clients as psychologically-complex individuals whilst simultaneously offering narrow, oversimplified and empirically-impoverished accounts of social realities. Moreover, seemingly iconoclastic calls for a revolution in our professional mindset turn out upon closer inspection to be merely re-hashed therapy-as-usual, tamely conservative at the level of understanding and intervention. I will suggest that the embrace of diversity by the therapy world has been warped by the need to shield our professional self-image and organisational structures from the crisis which a proper reckoning with diversity would entail. Current work on diversity risks discrediting a whole and very valuable area of inquiry. If a case is not made that these matters can be better addressed, some may wearily conclude that they just should not be talked of at all.

My argument is based on a close reading of recent UK-based academic and non-academic professional publications as well as workshop presentations I have attended. The problems I identify are typical of work in this area though inevitably the overall thrust of my criticism will map more fully onto some arguments than others. I will use the phrase 'diversity agenda' throughout the article to denote not merely a perceptible and dogmatic uniformity in assertion, but the way that diversity advocates aim at full professional support for a far-reaching program of action.

Diversity (ill-)defined

A term can only be defined as clearly as it is used; confused terminology can lead to confused thinking. At its most basic, the term diversity simply describes human variation. Descriptions often add a call for celebration: diversity is typically taken to be a good thing. Under the conceptual umbrella you will also find material on intercultural working and critical social justice (which takes the social fabric to be constituted primarily by insidious networks of power and privilege). Diversity is a kind of holophrase – a single term used in the service of multiple meanings – without possible inconsistency being acknowledged.

This linguistic compression erases important distinctions between different kinds of social phenomena, which require separate understanding. Cultural differences often require a quite different kind of comprehension than being a minority member of a majority culture (such as being gay) where a person might sometimes share in a majority mindset whilst differing at other times. Differences may be chosen or unavoidable, celebrated or regretted, permanent or transient. Too often discussions of the subject risk circling so far above the terrain that important distinctions disappear from view. We are more than capable of using different terms for meaningfully distinct phenomena and this would be a welcome development.

Why certain identity categories are deemed worthy of attention while others get passed over in silence is also contentious. At present race, sex/

gender and sexuality receive the most attention with the former very much first amongst equals at the time of writing. Dedicated concentration upon these categories comes perhaps less from self-evident clinical priorities than it does from their historic roots in venerable civil rights movements and their subsequent well-funded advocacy by dedicated academic disciplines and non-government organisations. Lacking alternative sources of knowledge upon which to draw, and almost certainly a little nervous about being branded prejudicial for failing to prioritise the needs of these high-profile groups, the therapy profession risks becoming a timorously deferential echo to the clamouring going on in the world at large. We forget at our peril that the loudest voices are not always the most representative.

Perhapsadvocates for these groups might claim that they are the ones most severely marked by oppression. In fact, there is abundant evidence that people of below average income, intelligence or attractiveness typically experience a range of comparable social disadvantages (Goodhart, 2020; Markovits, 2020; Minerva, 2017; Rhode, 2010). To date, workshops on 'counselling ugly people' are notable by their absence. Concluding that these groups have not organised politically because their difficulties are inconsequential is uncharitable. Failure to develop a collective political articulation of your predicament can be a sign of a more complete oppression, pernicious exactly because it is unnamed.

It would also help if affirmative and critical approaches to diversity were distinguished within our conversations. Celebrating diverse forms of life as different yet equal is sometimes incompatible with the need to acknowledge the inhibiting and deforming impact of oppression on collective identity formation. A previous generation of political thinkers (i.e. De Beauvoir & Rowbotham, 2009) argued that oppression had not merely put barriers in the way of otherwise fully-formed peoples, but that it left them incapable of conceiving how they would have been under non-oppressive circumstances. These arguments were necessary to explain that the present inferiority of certain groups was not a given. It is crucial to understand that whilst we may *celebrate* diversity, we are called upon to *abolish* oppression (see Michaels, 2006).

Diversity literature too often erases this distinction between the need for groups to not merely embrace who they are but *change* who they are because it is troubled by any gesture that appears to diminish people. Under the distal influence of the pervasive misappropriations of postmodern ideas, which proclaim the superiority of the marginalised (Cusset, 2008; Pluckrose & Lindsay, 2020), the diversity agenda wants to have it both ways. It claims that minority identity categories are both venerable and simultaneously formed by ubiquitous disadvantage. At first glance, this can seem a necessary group-level counterpart to our professional creed of respecting the dignity and worth of individuals. We must of course honour what remains of value in compromised lives, but if validation is not carefully qualified during the course of therapy it will encourage people to take their current limits for the horizon of their aspirations. Incompatible demands to name the ubiquity of oppression whilst celebrating all forms of life as equal can only be achieved by shrinking the scope of oppression down to minor disrespect by majority groups. Whilst the withholding of due estimation can indeed be painful, taking disrespect to be paradigmatic of oppression generally obscures more serious occurrences.

Our ethical requirement to recognise all group identities and cultures as equally valid also ultimately collides with the demand to understand important inter-group differences as structured by inequalities of power and privilege. It is hard to see how you can describe a social group as simultaneously oppressive towards others and also worthy of respect so we land by default on 'asymmetrical multiculturalism' (Kaufmann, 2018) where majority group cultures are denigrated and minority ones eulogised. No one has explained how therapists are supposed to treat majority population clients (male, white, heterosexual etc.) with the non-judgementalism necessary for good clinical work whilst also being compelled at other times to regard them as contemptable oppressors. Beginning from the premise that estimable and oppressive forms of diversity can exist concurrently in distinctive configurations within complex individual lives would surely be preferable.

Diversity in practice

As Russell Jacoby has shrewdly noted, the diversity agenda has the contradictory tendency to speak about a range of quite distinct phenomena in the same simplified way (Jacoby, 2020): the diversity agenda itself isn't very diverse! The plethora of writings and workshops currently in circulation are strikingly similar in phrasing and argumentative thrust. It can be reassuring when different authors reach the same conclusion independently because convergence can be taken to mean confirmation. Uniformity of expression is more concerning; to encounter the same narrow pool of ideas expressed in an interchangeable fashion again and again can leave us with the troubling impression that we are simply encountering the uncritical parroting of prominent ideas chosen without full awareness of the available alternatives. If there was a conversation in need of a greater range of informed voices engaging in open-minded discussion then it is this one.

More must be done about diversity, we are told, by writers who are thereby placing themselves ahead of other therapists designated by default as in need of moral instruction (Brown, 2005; Edwards, 2016; Jackson, 2017; Martin et al., 2020). Exhortations to be more 'courageous' (Holder, 2014) and to make oneself uncomfortable (Smith et al., 2021), frame any failure to concur with the author's preconceptions as resulting from a lack of nerve rather than a matter of constructive disagreement. Articles often feature supporting testimonies about the author's experiences of feeling overlooked, excluded and misunderstood in professional circles (Haghverdi et al., 2020).

Given that therapists are typically thoughtful people, generally left-leaning politically and who uncomplicatedly accept the aims of the diversity agenda, it is curious to encounter exhortations for them to embrace what they already believe. It is rarely clear what these authors think they are telling people that they don't already know when all they seem to be doing is repeating commonplace assumptions. It is also rare to see the author specify exactly what the 'more' is that they think everyone else should be doing except in the most abstract terms of 'more awareness', 'more sensitivity' etc. The notion of 'doing more' is by definition an ever-receding horizon. There is never a sense of what 'enough' might look like.

It is therefore not an uncommon experience to feel in discussions about diversity that an opportunity to inform has been squandered in favour of an opportunity to accuse. There is a clear parallel here between the ways in which diversity is presented within the profession and how it is often discussed outside. As more than one critic has noted (Fisher, 2013; McWhorter, 2021; Mitchell, 2022), there is a distinctively religious cast to some forms of contemporary identity politics which aims no higher than the recognition of hurt feelings and the enforced confession and the public denunciation of oppressors. This politics neither works towards increasing reconciliation between groups nor the practical solving of identified social problems, settling instead for the ritual hunting for heretics as a means of purifying the collective soul. Transfused into therapy trainings, this typically leads to discussions which are big on condemnation and short on increasing people's working knowledge and efficacy by giving them more precise conceptual tools and a firmer grasp of the relevant facts.

Therapy is a naturally hospitable to such practices since we already embrace a quasi-religious, confessional impetus to self-knowledge as a precondition of our work (Foucault, 1978). Yet just as contemporary identity politics can mistake the mere holding of righteous beliefs as synonymous with political efficacy (Lilla, 2018), so the therapy world sometimes treats the willingness and capacity for reflective self-exploration as the *only* precondition for an increased ability to work with diverse client groups (Basset, 2021). In doing so it collapses any meaningful distinction between reflexivity and learning. It is possible to be entirely unprejudiced towards a particular group whilst also being widely ignorant about them just as deep hostility towards a group can be found amongst people who are intimately familiar with them. The absence of prejudice is not synonymous with the presence of knowledge and there is a risk that inviting majority-population therapists to reflect upon their supposed biases will only ever end up promoting a majority view of what they take a minority group's typical experience to be. This well-intentioned gesture may ultimately end up misrepresenting minority voices in attempting to speak for them.

The most pernicious expression of this quasi-religious impulse can be found in workshops where stereotypic rituals of exploration, accusation and confession increasingly predominate. The elation which sometimes accompanies the act of confession can engender a false confidence that in exploring your own culpability so openly you become purified of ignorance. In a profession which valorises compassion and self-awareness, the suspicion that one has not done enough to demonstrate these virtues is a stain of dishonour. Participants entering diversity training usually understand the rules of the game well enough. They grasp that the encounter is already pre-scripted with privileged oppressors and the price of their penance presumptively named, weighed and assigned in advance. Many mouth the right words for fear that objection will simply be understood as confirmation of their unacknowledged bigotry (Church, 2020). The opportunity for honest exploration, encounter and learning is too often missed

The misunderstanding of oppression

Writing on diversity typically only acknowledges a problematically-narrow spectrum of oppression. There is a near-exclusive emphasis upon, to paraphrase Nancy Fraser (Fraser, 1997), relatively slight injuries of 'recognition' - interpersonal acts of othering, excluding, disrespect and shaming (Cameron, 2020; Turner, 2021). As I have argued elsewhere (Sedgwick, 2021) oppression more often aims at dominating (and exploiting) groups. Though by no means incompatible with injuries of recognition, domination is a quite distinct form of oppression which will not turn up in the same way in our client's stories, nor is it easily picked up by practitioners trained to think of psychological distress in relational terms.

Dominated populations are socially included but within a subordinate role, serving the interests of the dominating class. This oppression can be more distal, indirect and clandestine: it works best when the dominated don't notice exploitation is happening and don't believe that change is possible. It often operates through the omnipresent, unexamined presuppositions governing everyday life not just in negative interpersonal encounters. Dominated clients may be unable to name their oppression, act to alleviate it or hold their oppressors to account. There will often be a marked sense of confusion and defeat and a feeling that better worlds cannot be imagined. This kind of oppression plays little distinctive role in the literature on diversity.

It is a psychological precondition of experiencing rage and shame at minor indignities that a minority group must have already achieved a sufficient political awareness and sense of entitlement. Groups often move out of oppression unevenly and it is not uncommon for the more advantaged members to have needs and hopes which are quite distinct from those who lag behind. Therapists are often unaware that our ideas about the vulnerabilities of self-esteem to relational injuries have been quite self-consciously borrowed by some political movements to justify their claims to greater dignity in interpersonal matters (Lasch-Quinn, 2001). There is an identified tendency for relatively advantage members of a disadvantage group to treat their own needs as universally representative, to take control of political organisations and shape them in the service of their own relatively privileged interests (Reed, 2000; Táíwò, 2022). Redefining oppression to be mostly about minor misrecognitions typifies this manoeuvre. Therapists have been too credulous in accepting this because it is couched in language that is recognisably ours.

Respectful mention given to the dubious concept of 'microaggressions' (see Lilianfeld, 2017) therefore represents not the belated discovery of new oppressions but the naïve redefinition of the concept in terms of slight examples. Microaggressions are a mostly inconsequential part of life for many people, particularly in societies run along market lines where competition and meritocracy leave many struggling for status. I am not claiming that seemingly minor insults never have great personal significance. It is precisely a hallmark of good therapeutic practice that we attend respectfully to what things mean for our clients without worrying about how they might be typically experienced by others. I'm simply pointing out that in the effort not to further harm minority group clients, we can falsely presume that relatively slight experiences of misrecognition are always and everywhere hurtful in the same way: in doing so, we replace our customary professional respect for varied, psychological complexity with an insistence upon uniform psychological fragility.

In our fear of underestimating the insidious reach and impact of prejudice, we can end up misrepresenting whole groups as brittle by definition. By inference, those quickest to injure and first to speak are taken to be best placed to voice the collective group experience. This creates an inverted hierarchy which valorises suffering over coping. Sweeping definitions of entire groups as always vulnerable discounts the many individuals who have triumphed in the face of adversity or endured prejudice without being defined by it. My own experiences suggest that many clients are unhappy that their diversity-sensitive therapist has prematurely ghettoised them into an identity category and presumed their fragility by insisting that tolerated experiences are actually grievous emotional wounds whose significance they are downplaying. The silencing of such voices is just another consequence of diversity's reductive homogeneity.

Advocates of the diversity agenda also tend to paint an oversimplified picture of social context. Analysis is conducted using a handful of facts and a limited palate of concepts, most often 'power' and 'privilege' though terms like 'systemic' and 'structural' are now appearing with increasing regularity

(Beetham, 2019). When used properly these concepts can be a useful means for understanding some aspects our client's social realities, yet it often seems as if the author is using them solely for a kind of aesthetic effect. It as though mere citation might provide a patina of conceptual gravitas and technical know-how to arguments that might otherwise sound rather unconvincing were they more plainly stated. We are offered merely the vocabulary of critique without its substance.

Successful critique presupposes immanence; it must begin from an empirically-rich sense of *how* things are as a starting point for uncovering *why* things are as they are (Habermas, 1988). Having shown why things are as they are, it points the way to a better state of affairs. The term power is rarely defined in diversity literature and almost always used in a way which departs from its typical definition as the capacity to get others to do something against their will or interests (Lukes, 2005). Used well, the concept of power enhances critical understanding and identifies options for action. Looking away from the relatively inconsequential micropower of personal encounters towards institutional, statutory and legislative mechanisms would represent a genuine advance, but even here critical ideas must be combined with a detailed grasp of social specifics. If authors are going to talk about systems and structures they need to present a fuller account of exactly what they are referring to, their internal mechanisms and the nature of their impact. Instead, we too often get barely-supported generalisations about a group's collective experience or individual stories offered up as representative. The former typically descends into catastrophizing and cliché; the later cannot overcome the inevitable objection that individual stories don't always represent collective experience.

Clinical work requires an empiricallyrich understanding of social factors and typical group experience sufficient to illuminate the specific manifestations of general social conditions applying to a particular client. Done properly, knowledge of what is socially typical will not detract from our understanding of the individual but enhance it. If we can understand our client's stories as distally structured by multiple, varying and sometimes contradictory instances of power, ebbing and flowing in the course of their daily existence which makes certain actions and thoughts more or less likely, more or less achievable as the person moves through the world, then we will have achieved something usefully precise which can inform clinical work. Understanding the participants in a therapeutic dyad in terms of a static, standardised portion of power and privilege based on a simplistic picture of their respective group memberships is not enough. Replacing unknowing open-mindedness with crude stereotyping is not progress.

Basing our clinical work on simple, dystopian fairy tales about the world does not merely mis-represent it also misdirects. It risks plunging struggling clients into a state of unnecessary paranoia and pessimism under the false promise of naming their unacknowledged hurt to better heal it (Boltanski, 2011). We name power to help our clients spot it, side-step it, gain more of it or take it away from those who wield it against them. It is not just another means of identifying yet more injuries of recognition to be met empathically. It's a sorry state of affairs when a profession that insists upon understanding a client's inner world in the highest possible fidelity is simultaneously so easily satisfied with an oversimplification of those same client's outer worlds. Psychological nuance is disregarded in a rush to place clients within a crudely sketched social firmament. This may often be worse than not considering questions of diversity at all.

The underlying rationale for the diversity agenda

The many difficulties identified here result indirectly from unacknowledged problems in our professional self-understanding and organisation. When I deliver training on the social context of distress I note that participants invariably turn up excepting to hear standard diversity fare about injuries of recognition in racial and sexual minorities. My efforts to persuade them that the most important difficulties typically facing certain groups are not injuries of recognition and therefore might not benefit from a relational conceptualisation often do not please them. Participants arrive hoping to extended but not change their working practices. They clearly hope to be told what they already know.

The diversity agenda has spread so quickly throughout the profession not merely because of its wider cultural ubiquity but because of its self-conscious deployment of therapeutic ideas. If you are told that what matters most are injuries of recognition in daily interactions then you are already embracing a vision of diversity which fits snugly inside an unmodified version of your therapeutic model's core relational assumptions which you use for all clients anyway. If all you are trained to look for is injuries of recognition then those are the only things you are going to find.

Minority-group therapists protesting their thoughtless misunderstanding at the hands of their colleagues may fancy themselves to be insurgent outsiders but they are actually attacking the profession on its own preferred terms. Accuser and accused are united in unthinking deference to their chosen relational assumptions and professional skill-set. That relational approaches to clinical work might not be the best way to understand or respond to certain forms of disadvantage is therefore never considered. Everyone in the conversation is predisposed to keep something like therapy-as-usual on its pedestal. The possibility of a more radical or materially-rooted approach to clinical work, or something other than therapy entirely such as practical help, political action or consciousness-raising, is therefore never raised.

Effective work with diverse and disadvantaged client groups customarily requires an immersive familiarity with their forms of life in addition to general clinical knowhow. As a middle-class man practicing in areas of high social and economic deprivation, it has taken many years of careful, reflective learning for this necessary knowledge to appear. I don't believe there are always short-cuts and I'm troubled that the diversity agenda seems to promise them. There is an assumption that 'working with cultural difference' and, say, 'working with anxiety' are somehow similar learning tasks when they are quite different in both nature and scope. The latter can be done briefly by learning a set of general working principles which are applied with variation to fit individual cases. The former is rather like learning to speak in a new language. It entails extended, respectful immersion in a form of life until its unique internal logic, its history and its cadences are intuitively grasped.

I have spent most of my working life as part of a team where it was often possible to match a client with a practitioner who understood their part of the world, yet we typically conceive of therapists as lone practitioners trained to see a full spectrum of clients. The most obvious reason for this is that teams of therapists possessing the kind of immersive familiarity with particular communities necessary for effective work would have to be planned, recruited and funded with state support. I believe moving towards specialist organisations based around targeted recruitment is a material and organisational precondition for addressing some of the concerns I have raised so far. The problem is both that we lack the current means to make this happen and fencing off large areas of work as requiring immersive life experience may be particularly unpopular with private practitioners whose revenue streams in a competitive marketplace presume minimal limits on the kinds of clients they can see.

The hasty embrace of the diversity agenda therefore heads off a serious challenge to our professional self-image since it prevents us from acknowledging that the usual tripartite division of theoretical mastery, personal development and clinical experience are necessary and sufficient conditions for producing complete practitioners. Take diversity seriously and you have to admit advanced social awareness of particular forms of life as an additional requirement. This may be why the diversity agenda doesn't just flatter our preferred modalities by focusing on injuries of recognition, it also says how we usually work doesn't need to change much. We are selling therapists on the idea that diversity competence can be spooned-out at half-day workshops offering stereo-typed depictions of group experience and accompanied by redemptive confessions of power and privilege. Given the pressure to do something, can we blame people for participating in a reassuring pretence of adequacy as they wait to collect their certificates after the lunch-time samosas have been served?

Meeting the challenges that diversity poses will require both improved conceptual tools and professional reorganisation that can support grassroots knowledge production. Focusing solely on the former at the expense of the latter will yield only partial gains. Without an open acknowledgement of the nature and scale of the problem we face the diversity agenda will stumble onwards, magnifying small hurts and ignoring larger ones, mistaking confessions of privilege for the acquisition of useful knowledge, claiming to be radically reforming our practice whilst at the same implying that nothing much needs to change and offering only a thin, emollient illusion of competence which evaporates upon contact with the unforgiving realities of clinical practice.

Note

1. For the purpose of this article I will use the generic term therapy to cover counselling and psychotherapy.

Disclosure statement

No potential conflict of interest was reported by the author.

References

Basset, F. (2021). Members accounts/inclusion in psychotherapy. *New Psychotherapist*, *77* (2), 45.
Beetham, T. (2019, April 18–19). Intersectionality and social justice. *Therapy Today*.
Boltanski, L. (2011). *On critique: A sociology of emancipation* (G. Elliot, Trans.). Polity.
Brown, C. (2005, September 20). Letter – Diversity matters. *Therapy Today*.
Cameron, R. (2020). *Working with difference and diversity in counselling and psychotherapy*. Sage.
Church, J. D. (2020). *Reinventing racism: Why "White Fragility" is the wrong way to think about racial inequality*. Rowman & Littlefield Publishers.
Cusset, F. (2008). *French theory: How Foucault, Derrida, Deleuze, & Co. transformed the intellectual life of the United States* (J. Fort, J. Berganza, & M. Jones, Trans.). U of Minnesota Press.
Dalal, F. (2008). Against the celebration of diversity. *British Journal of Psychotherapy*, *24*(1), 4–19. https://doi.org/10.1111/j.1752-0118.2007.00060.x
De Beauvoir, S., & Rowbotham, S. (2009). *The second sex* (C. Borde & S. Malovny-Chevalier, Trans.). Vintage.
Edwards, P. (2016). Letter to the editor - Confronting internalised racism. *Therapy Today*, *27*(8), 34.
Fisher, M. (2013, November 22). Exiting the vampire castle. *The North Star*. https://www.opendemocracy.net/en/opendemocracyuk/exiting-vampire-castle/

Foucault, M. (1978). *The history of sexuality, vol. 1: The will to knowledge* (R. Hurley, Trans.). Penguin.

Fraser, N. (1997). *Justice interruptus: Critical reflections on the 'postsocialist' condition.* Routledge.

Goodhart, D. (2020). *Head hand heart: The struggle for dignity and status in the 21st century.* Penguin UK.

Habermas, J. (1988). *On the logic of the social sciences* (S. W. Nicholsen & J. A. Stark, Trans.). Polity Press.

Haghverdi, J., Williamson, A., Benjamin, A., Mason, N., Adenekan, L., & Shaheen-Zaffar, Y. (2020). Race in the room: How do we change the narrative around racism and really start to listen to each other. *Therapy Today, 31*(8), 24–26.

Holder, J. (2014). We need courageous conversations. *Therapy Today, 25*(8), 33.

Jackson, C. (2017). Putting gender on the agenda. *Therapy Today, 28*(10), 8–11.

Jacoby, R. (2020). *On diversity: The eclipse of the individual in a global era.* Seven Stories.

Kaufmann, E. (2018). *White shift: Population, immigration and the future of white majorities.* Penguin.

Lasch-Quinn, E. (2001). *Race experts: How racial etiquette, sensitivity training, and new age therapy hijacked the civil rights revolution.* WW Norton & Co.

Lilianfeld, S. O. (2017). Microaggressions: Strong claims, inadequate evidence. *Perspectives on Psychological Science, 12*(1), 138–169. https://doi.org/10.1177/1745691616659391

Lilla, M. (2018). *The once and future liberal: After identity politics.* Hurst & Co.

Lukes, S. (2005). *Power: A radical approach* (2nd ed.). Red Globe.

Markovits, D. (2020). *The meritocracy trap.* Penguin.

Martin, B., Paine, M., Christopher, J., & Halacre, M. (2020). Addressing our racism. *Therapy Today, 31*(8), 12–13.

McWhorter, J. (2021). *Woke racism: How a new religion has betrayed black America.* Penguin books.

Michaels, W. B. (2006). *The trouble with diversity: How we learned to love identity and ignore inequality.* Metropolitan Books.

Minerva, F. (2017). The invisible discrimination before our eyes: A bioethical analysis. *Bioethics, 31*(3), 180–189. https://doi.org/10.1111/bioe.12327

Mitchell, J. (2022). *American awakening: Identity politics and other afflictions of our time.* Encounter Books.

Pluckrose, H., & Lindsay, J. (2020). *Cynical theories: How activist scholarship made everything about race, gender and identity – and why this harms everyone.* Pitchstone Publishing.

Reed, A., Jr. (2000). *Class notes: Posing as politics and other thoughts on the American scene.* The New Press.

Rhode, D. L. (2010). *The beauty bias: The injustice of appearance in life and law.* Oxford University Press.

Sedgwick, J. M. (2021). *Contextual transactional analysis: The inseparability of self and world.* Routledge.

Smith, L., Proctor, G., & Akondo, D. (2021). Confronting racism in counselling and therapy training—Three experiences of a seminar on racism and whiteness. *Psychotherapy & Politics International, 19*(2), 1–11. https://doi.org/10.1002/ppi.1579

Táíwò, O. O. (2022). *Elite capture: How the powerful took over identity politics (and everything else).* Pluto.

Turner, D. W. (2021). *Intersections of privilege and otherness in counselling and psychotherapy.* Routledge.

A psychotherapist's lived experience in-session with an asylum seeker and translator: An autoethnographic case study

Nicole Chew-Helbig

ABSTRACT

Featured in this article is a psychotherapy case study recounted from the lived experience of the psychotherapist working with an asylum seeker from Afghanistan, with the help of a translator. The method applied is an aesthetic inquiry adapted from Autoethnography which engages the practitioner as the researcher who enters the 'field' of the therapy situation. The reflexive writing of the case story, which is integral to the method, sets off a heuristic process, integrating research and practice. Reading this case study, one may grasp the nuances and the atmosphere of an otherwise linguistically challenging therapeutic situation. The story and Gestalt therapy theory are weaved together, which makes palpable, intangible aspects of the therapeutic process.

Introduction

Presented here is a psychotherapy case study of a psychotherapist's phenomenological experience of working with a client, an asylum seeker, with the assistance of a translator. Autoethnography is the method applied to this study. While the application of Autoethnography to psychotherapy research exists (Grant, 2010; Jones, 2015; Siddique, 2011; Talbot, 2018), the approach used here, and a recent writing (Chew-Helbig, 2022), is differentiated by 1) applying the method to inquiry into psychotherapy process, 2) defining the therapist as autoethnographer, and 3) defining the therapeutic encounter as the field. The product of Autoethnography is the aesthetic form of writing, a creative non-fiction.

This method promises to help us grasp the non- and pre-verbal nuances, the aesthetic aspect of the therapeutic situation, of the psychotherapy process and psychopathology that current research paradigms grapple with. Theory and practice are then integrated by weaving in story with theory. Demonstrated here is a possibility, through the method, for therapists to exchange naturalistic in-practice learnings.

Method

Autoethnography, defined in Adams et al. (2015) and Poulos (2021), is a qualitative research method, that delivers a genre of academic writing that is evocative, reflexive, creative and aesthetic. This aesthetic inquiry belongs to a post-modernistic attitude towards research.

The method positions the psychotherapist as autoethnographer. The 'field' is the therapy process of a client being studied. Data is derived from the practitioner's session notes, which are also the field notes. Autoethnography is an observational, data-driven phenomenological method. When used to study a client's psychotherapeutic process from the viewpoint of the practitioner, invaluable phenomenological insights can be obtained. Integral to the process of doing this research is its reflexive writing. We use theory to inquire and explain the nuances of experience, while the story is a mechanism that illustrates how these nuances are sensed and felt (Adams et al., 2015, p. 90). Both theory and story exist symbiotically, and in this article, are presented together.

Actors in this case study are: 1) the client, Ali,[1] who's about 30. He arrived in Vienna from Afghanistan 3 months earlier and was seeking asylum status in Vienna. He was referred to the clinic by social services, having been diagnosed with posttraumatic stress disorder (PTSD). 2) The therapist, who's in her late 40s, is Singaporean and has lived in Austria for more than a decade. She is a Gestalt therapist in private practice, and the narrator of this case study. 3) The translator, Zaya, who is in her early 40s, is Iranian, and was training as a therapist, and was on a student's visa in Vienna.

Case study: 'Undercurrent'

Zaya, the translator for our sessions, was already there when I entered the spacious therapy room of the psychotherapy clinic in Vienna. There is a cardboard file on the coffee table in front of her with its documents spewed out.

It is a chilly autumn morning and the air in the room has not warmed up yet. In the corridor outside the room, are sounds of other colleagues getting started for the day. In about fifteen minutes we expect the client, Ali, to walk in. We look silently through Ali's file. A little bit of preparation can calm nerves. 'Sometimes they don't want to come', says Zaya, who has already translated for many Farsi-speaking clients. Ali is the first client from the asylum seeker group that I am being assigned to. I find support in Zaya's words. Yes. I can imagine how many who are living in the camps would not like to come for therapy, especially so early in the morning. Then there's Ali who is a man shy of thirty. He has fled his home in Kabul a couple of months before. He is probably one of thousands of asylum seekers now fearing possible deportation. What could possibly motivate him to sit in this room in therapy with two women who are almost a generation older than he is? Putting Ali's intake questionnaires together with the diagnostic reports back into the file, I thank her for being here.

By the time Ali walked in, we were both leaning back on chairs arranged around the little glass coffee table. Ali takes his seat on the empty chair. He keeps his puffed bomber jacket on.

***

I have been wary of the prospect of having a translator in the therapy room, concerned about having to form a connection with the client while relying on a go-between, whose presence could potentially feel like a kind of interference. A part of me has lent myself to the opinion of many colleagues who do not want to face this experience. The other part of me is curious about the process.

Ali settles himself down. He has a head of unkempt curly hair, his smile, cherubic. He smiles a lot. Ali and I share a silent smile and a nod. He exchanges some words with Zaya that sound like casual greetings.

> 'Here we are', I start, 'three of us'.
> Zaya translates.

With this first turn, I feel a warmth. Zaya's presence is a support that fills a certain void between me and the client. I'm also painfully aware of how this sensation of being supported feels long-lost. The translator in the session listens intently to every word we say. She echoes the phrases in her mother tongue, a language that is totally foreign to me. She lends herself no voice of her own. I pendulate between feeling thankful and awkward. Am I speaking too quickly? Am I not sufficiently coherent? I shrug off thoughts that I am burdening the translator. I notice myself feeling responsible for everyone else in the room.

***

On the phenomenological experience of pathos

Prior to entering the field, the therapist had an expectation of working with a translator in the session, having taken reference from other colleagues. On contact with the field, she was touched by an experience that felt alien to her. Francesetti (2019) describes the experience of being moved beyond our ability to make logic out of the experience, is described as the *pathic*. 'We are seized by the pathic; we do not choose it, we are moved by it; pathic has the same root as passion and pathology, both happen to us and take us without choice: it is something *to which* we are subject (rather than *of which* we are subject)' (Francesetti, 2019, p. 41). The therapist sensed this suffering, though it was not made explicit at the time of the session. In a phenomenological field, experiences are allowed to emerge, which are not merely subjective reality, but also unique to the moment, ephemeral, co-created, situated, corporeal and dynamic. Even though the pathos described here is felt by, and belongs to the therapist, it belongs to the field of the triad as well.

***

The client, Ali, as reflected in his intake documents, is diagnosed with PTSD. He arrived in Austria having bought his way out of Afghanistan by paying human smugglers to take him, along with a group of other Afghani men, on a treacherous passage by land that lasted months. In Austria, he was homed in a remote Austrian village, from which he absconded, ending up in a camp in Vienna. While he awaits getting his asylum status approved in Vienna, he is provided with lodging, a payout of about 800 Euros per month, and a middle high school education. Until Ali's asylum status is approved, he lives with the possibility of being deported back to Afghanistan. Zaya and I are acutely mindful of the immense stress this uncertainty – over and above the other imminent issues – can have, as this is part of the ongoing discourse surrounding all of us who work with asylum seekers.

In these first moments of meeting Ali, I notice myself fighting (and then accepting) within me, a sensation of dread; my limbs feel heavy, my breathing shallow. I sense shifts of fearing not being of use as a therapist for the client and burdening the translator, to fearing feeling the pain of getting to know a client who may go through deportation.

> 'I want to be understood', says Ali, still smiling, when I asked what he would like to have happen for him through our work together. 'I want to achieve things'.
> Zaya translates.
> 'I would like that for myself too, to be understood and to achieve things', I say,
> Zaya translates.
> There's cautious laughter.
> 'I'm wondering, what are the things you wish to achieve?' I ask.
> Zaya translates.
> 'Things. Like I am scared of saying "hello" to Anna'. He replies, and grins; a teenager revealing a crush.
> Zaya translates.
> 'Anna', I smile back.
> Zaya smiles.
> 'Anna', says Ali.

Pre-formation of the contact

The awareness of the ongoing phenomena that emerges from background of the field brings about an opportunity for making contact with the environment, the atmosphere, the pathos. Through this contact, pathological states can then be actualized, assimilated and melt back into the background, in an awareness continuum (Yontef, 1993, p. 139).

The information written in the intake documents consists of reports of 'facts'. The therapist's reaction to the content of the client's documents is a feeling of dread. This feeling belongs to the therapist in isolation. The moment the therapist and client make contact, is the pre-formation of the contact. It is where the perceptive experience of the other is undifferentiated, diffused, and yet to emerge. The therapist describes a point where she, and perhaps the others of the field, finds herself seized by feelings of uneasiness of the yet unknown, and very-soon-to-be-experienced emerging convergence of fields.

***

> *'I want to be confident, but something in my past is stopping me', Zaya translates.*

I give Ali a nod to acknowledge what I am hearing. He smiles back at me. His jacket hangs on a clothes rack by the door. This is the start of our second session.

Ali's opening sentence this morning feels like an invitation. Ali stands by a threshold between the future and the past. He points us in the direction of the past. I see him shudder. I shudder, though I do not know what it is I am seeing. I am interested, in earnest. I am also wary. I lean back.

***

Field perspective of psychopathology

The client repeats his desire for moving on into the future, and says, '*but something in my past is stopping me*'. He repeats this in his first two sessions and several sessions thereafter. I tend to see the client's initial utterance as their attempt at being present with their pathos, making it palpable to the therapist. By responding to the pathos in the field (Francesetti, 2015), the therapist supports the emergence of the client's self, and his suffering in the field.

Responding to the sensed pathos in the field is potentially more useful to the therapist than a DSM (American Psychiatric Association, 2013) diagnosis. The diagnosis of PTSD written in the client's documents provided little for the therapist to use. A DSM diagnosis is mono-personal, relevant to the client in isolation, while the pathological field belongs to the client with the therapist in the situation of their encounter. The mono-personal approach to diagnosis, a dominant paradigm of psychiatry and the DSM, focuses the treatment of symptoms experienced by the individual, while the bi-personal approach of relational modalities of psychotherapy affirms therapeutic change to arise through the therapeutic alliance (BCPSG, 2010; Clarkson, 2003; Greenberg, 1986; Jacobs & Hycner, 2009). Attunement to the aesthetics of the pathological field promises to expand the practitioner's reach even further. The field perspective challenges us to view psychotherapy as a convergence of the inter-subjective field of the therapist and the client and an emergence of a phenomenological (or pathological) field. Theory of the field is central to Gestalt therapy (Parlett, 1991; Philippson, 2009; Staemmler, 2006) as it is in psychology (Lewin, 1951). The field forms the holistic organization of the individuals of the therapeutic situation. The therapist, client, and translator find themselves in contact, and passively subjected to, the phenomenon of this field, which is characteristically emergent, unique, ephemeral, situated, co-created, corporeal, and dynamic.

***

I ask Ali what he meant by the past stopping him from being confident.

'Uncle'. Ali explains that uncle is the younger brother of his father. Ali was put in the care of uncle and his wife when he was 9 years old. Till he turned 18, Ali lived with the couple and their daughter, who's a little younger than Ali. 'I always hear uncle say, "you will come to nothing. Nothing"'.

> 'What would you say to him right now, if he is sitting here?' I ask.
> Zaya translates.
> Ali clenches a fist, then promptly holds it down with the other hand. 'I have no words, nothing'.
> 'Yes'. I say. I give space to the young man's rage. Zaya reaches gingerly for a filled paper cup and takes a sip. Ali and I follow suit.
> I ask him how he got to be put in the care of uncle.

'After school I play football. The playground is near my house. One day, I was playing football, then the bomb of the Taliban exploded on our house'. Zaya translates this, ice cold. They were all home when it happened; Ali's father Zabi, his mother, Fatemeh and his baby sister Khatere. Ali's voice cracks as he mentions the name of his baby sister. He stares, glassy-eyed, blank.

The skin on the back of my neck tingles. I glance towards the radiator by the window, as if to check if it was turned on properly. No, the air in the room is not cold. I am being touched by phantoms who have now descended amongst us. I search my bag for paper, only to find a dog-eared stack of neon coloured post-its. I write, 'Zabi', 'Fatemeh', 'Khatere', on three little sheets, careful to get the spelling right. I lay the post-its on the coffee table. I feel tears well up in my eyes. The space between us is saturated.

***

Creative indifference and the fertile void

Creative indifference is a term coined by German-Jewish philosopher and satirist, Salomo Friedländer (born 1871). The original German term for 'creative' is *schöpferische*, to 'create' in a way God creates, which is different from the meaning of having something made up. To be *indifferent*, refers to being intentionally disinterested, impartial, unbiased. It is important to qualify that being *disinterested* is the contrast of being *uninterested*, which is apathy. *Apathy* is the flattening of experience, the falling asleep to the pathos. Creative indifference embraces the possibility of diverse phenomena, that allows the therapist to be present to, and in contact with, the client's pathological field with open curiosity. In German, the term used by Friedländer is, *das Weltenschwangere Nichts*, which means literally, 'the nothingness that gives birth to worlds' (Frambach, 2003). This nothingness is also referred to as the fertile void.

There are many ways of explaining the concept of Creative Indifference. In this example, it is the virtue of patience, of taking time for the void of not-knowing to happen; by slowing down the conversation, by bringing attention to the emptiness of the space. In that space an uneasiness is felt by all. In holding this space, the therapist supports the client in sharing a wounded part of his childhood. All who were present experienced the pathos, the grief, that the client, at that moment, no longer was alone with.

***

'How … are … you?' Ali asks me in English, then giggles.
'Thank you, Ali', I say. 'I slept well, so this morning you have my fullest attention'.
Zaya translates.
'How about you, Zaya', I ask.
I catch a slight blush in her cheeks, as she giggles, 'very well'.
'Ali says that he doesn't sleep well. For example last night he had a bad dream. A nightmare'. Zaya translates.

'There is the mafia', Ali says, 'who is raiding the castle. Me and my friends are hiding in it. The mafia shoots me. I'm almost dying and my friends save me. My father is there. Oh. But that is only for a short time. I fall out of the window and run away'.

We share a round of chuckling. I offer Ali and Zaya a suggestion to do a chair work. Zaya's eyes lights up. I'm aware that she had read much about the Gestalt therapy method of working with dreams. 'I'm not sure if you'd like to try this exercise'. I say to Ali, who is probably sensing Zaya's interest.

'Yes. Yes', is his reply.
'Well, if at any time either of you are feeling unwell doing this dreamwork, say stop'. I tell them.
'Yes. Yes', he says.
Zaya translates, 'What do I do?'

So we set the stage with empty chairs around us. I am thankful for having booked this larger room again this morning. Ali puts a chair for 'the mafia' a distant right from his. He then says that the rows of chairs stacked up along the wall of the room are where his friends sit. He takes the last chair and places it close behind him slightly to his left; there Ali seats his father.

This is the dreamwork, abridged (see Figure 1)

Interspersed within the dialogue is the translation process.

Therapist: 'We are all seated together in Ali's dream. The mafia sits on this chair to your right, and your father is sitting behind you to your left. Zaya and I are sitting in front of your friends. How is this for you?'

Ali: 'I don't want to talk to the mafia. The mafia is inhuman, does things that humans will not do'.

Therapist: 'What would you need to tell the mafia?'

Ali: 'To be more human'.

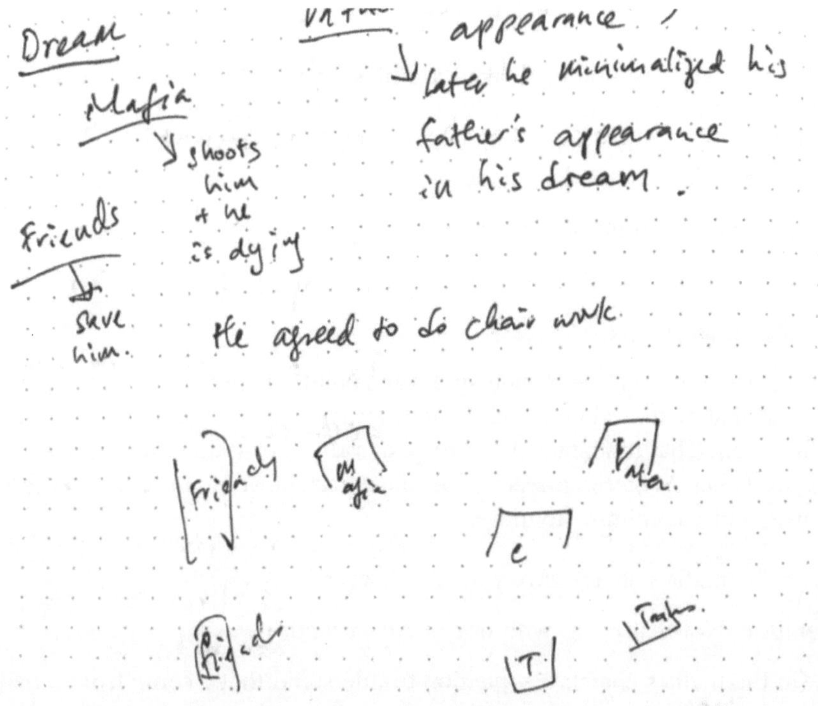

Figure 1. Excerpt from the therapist notes describing the dreamwork.

Therapist: 'How would the mafia answer to what you have just said?'

Ali shrugs.

I invite Ali to play the mafia, perhaps by sitting on the empty chair of the mafia.

Ali: 'No, no'.

Therapist: 'Then, should we ask the mafia to go away?'

Ali: 'No, no. Mafia can stay'.

Therapist: 'There is a chair behind you. Who sits there?'

Ali turns around, looks at the chair and turns back.

Ali: 'He was only there for a short while, in the beginning'.

Therapist: 'Your father. He was not there for very long'.

Ali: 'Yes'.

Therapist: 'How do you feel about your father sitting behind you?'

Ali: 'I feel good. But he's only here for a short time'.

Therapist: 'Yes'.

At this point, I would have liked to linger on with having a conversation with Ali's father, but I notice Ali's attention drift to the chair of the mafia. He turns to look at the chair of the mafia. I check with him what he was experiencing looking at that chair.

Ali: 'I am not so afraid of him (the mafia) now'.

Therapist: 'What has changed?'

Ali: 'My father is here'.

Ali shakes his head side-to-side, smiles and points to the chair, as if asking if it was okay that he moved to that chair now. He rises up and seats himself on the mafia's chair. That moment, I felt a tinge of sadness of seeing him move away from his father. My feelings seem to be in contrast, however, to Ali's mood. He has just motivated himself to move.

Ali (in the mafia's chair): 'Are you Ali's lawyer?'

Therapist: 'Not really. I'm with one of Ali's friends'.

Ali (in the mafia's chair): 'People don't understand that I come from a bad place where I have to do these things'.

I am aware that the session is almost up, and decide at this moment not to ask what 'these things' are.

Therapist to translator: 'I'm thinking that Ali looks a little different, sitting in this chair right now. What do you observe?'

Translator: 'Umm. A little. Umm. Yes'.

Therapist: 'What is different, do you reckon?'

Translator: 'Ali's no longer squeezing his hands together, he is sitting straight, he looks serious, not smiling as much'.

Time is up for the session. Ali says that he would like to stay in the mafia's chair till the end. 'It might help me with my school exams next week', Zaya translates.

We sit in this constellation for a while, in silence. Though not able to really grasp the meaning of this moment, I feel the lightness of gratitude.

***

Gestalt therapy dreamwork

The above example is one of several methods of working with dreams in Gestalt therapy. This one is where the dream is acted out. In the dreamwork, the therapist brings the dream of the client into the space of the room with the use of empty chairs. The entire atmosphere is felt. From the work above, we observe how latent contents of the dream (Freud, 1899/1995), which are projected parts of the client's personality manifested as characters in the dream, are invited to show up in the therapy room.

> Freud once called the dream the Via Regia, the royal road to the unconscious. And I believe it is really the royal road to integration . . . The dream is the most spontaneous expression of the existence of the human being. (Perls, 1969/1992, p. 87)

***

The first sessions had set the aesthetics – the atmosphere – of the field, a meeting of three erstwhile (seemingly) discreet individuals, and the connecting of our phenomenological/pathological fields. Through the connection, we realize our own pathos; not only that of the client.

'My life is like the sea', says Ali six months into our work together, 'top is calm, underneath is in turmoil'. Ali uses this metaphor to impress on us how he yearns to be happy, but is haunted by the past, and that he is plagued by feelings of remorse for what he has done. He has also become aware of his feelings of envy towards the local citizens of Vienna. Being amongst the privileged of this European city, he painfully reminds himself of how fate has robbed him of the dignified life that seems to belong so naturally to others.

Listening to Ali's articulate expression of his experience today – words that are still being translated to me by Zaya – I am filled with admiration. Not only for the client, but for everyone of us in this field. The Ali sitting in this room this morning looks very much an adult. He no longer wears his hair in tousled curls, having shaven them off 2 weeks ago. His face is also no longer smiley-cherubic, but sad and thoughtful. Lately, we share some words in German. This is the session where I am also painfully aware that our final session is near.

Zaya has tears in her eyes. I ask her if she's aware of an emotion she's feeling. 'Grief', she replies. I allow the word to settle upon us and give space for Zaya to compose herself, before moving on.

After the session ended, and we're both alone together, Zaya breaks down in tears. The pathos of this morning's session has filled her with deep feelings of grief. It was Ali's metaphor of the sea. She has, in recent months, lost two friends in separate situations to drowning – a schoolmate of her own child, and a good friend living in Iran, a young father of three – both violently swept away by currents beneath calm waters. I'm reminded of my friend, Ash. We sat together for a while. I couldn't contain my tears.

We gathered for nine months, three months longer than we had contracted to work together. In this field, a story and plot emerged. Ali's plot toggles between contents of his past and his future. From the former we hear of his suicide attempts, the violent treatment he endured from his uncle, the friends he had lost in the war. We hear of his concern for the women he had left behind in Afghanistan who had protected him – his uncle's wife, and the mother of his friend, also named Ali. We hear also of betrayal. Ali's future promises hope, despair, and uncertainty. What we had together was in the here-and-now, like a pivot, holding space in an undifferentiated situation.

Discussion

In working with disenfranchised groups, witnesses of oppression and violence, being present to their pain has far reaching effects on the much wider field. Violence is the transference of pain that is absent in the perpetrator to the victim. Pain is transferred until it is transformed (Weil, 1952). In the therapeutic encounter, that transformation can happen, transcending language and culture. This brings us full circle to the value of tuning in to aesthetics in psychotherapy research – through autoethnography – and practice – through attunement to the atmosphere of the field. *Aesthetics* is derived from the Greek origin of 'the sense of perception'. Contrast this with the *an-aesthetics* of medical science, and we may be able to appreciate the difference in the understanding of psychopathology and treatment of pain in both fields. The client who is suffering usually describes themselves as being depressed, dissociated and numb. Psychopathological suffering is in essence an absence, rather than the pain itself (Francesetti, 2012). In the case story above, the client repeats that *something* in his past was keeping him from moving on. That *something* is a hint at the pathos. When the therapist becomes present to the client's pathos, they become present to suffering that was, till then, suffered alone by a nine-year-old child. This experience of being with the client, could have been missed had we settled with clinical diagnostics. The inquiry into the clients' suffering, is psychopathology that is an integral and effective part of the therapeutic process.

Current gaps in the field of psychotherapy research, according to Lutz et al. (2021, p. 11), involve the understanding of change processes in diverse, naturalistic psychotherapy environments, which remain ungraspable despite decades of quantitative, and even current qualitative research methods. This case study provides us the possibility to address the issue of communicating the aesthetic, and for the practitioner to contribute to this knowledge base. There is a heuristic aspect (Moustakas, 1990) of this process, a never-ending hermeneutic loop of understanding the therapeutic process and psychopathology. Using this research methodology alone, however, offers limited possibility of providing the objective and quantifiable data, which is still the predominant scientific paradigm.

Note

1. All the actors, and characters mentioned are given pseudonyms.

Disclosure statement

No potential conflict of interest was reported by the author.

ORCID

Nicole Chew-Helbig http://orcid.org/0000-0003-2649-7329

References

Adams, T., Jones, S. H., & Ellis, C. (2015). *Autoethnography: Understanding qualitative research*. Oxford.

American Psychiatric Association. (2013). *DSM-5. Diagnostic and statistical manual of mental disorders*. APA.

BCPSG. (2010). *Change in psychotherapy*. W. W. Norton & Co.

Chew-Helbig. (2022). Writing evocative case studies: Applying autoethnography as a research methodology for the psychotherapist. *The British Gestalt Journal, 31*(1), 35–42.

Clarkson, P. (2003). *The therapeutic relationship*. Whurr Publishers.

Frambach, L. (2003). The weighty world of nothingness: Salomo Friedlaender's *creative indifference*. In M. Spagnuolo Lobb & N. Armendt-Lyon (Eds.), *Creative license. The art of Gestalt therapy* (pp. 113–128). Springer.

Francesetti, G. (2012). Pain and beauty: From the psychopathology to the aesthetics of contact. *British Gestalt Journal, 21*(2), 4–18.

Francesetti, G. (2015). From individual symptoms to psychopathological fields. Towards a field perspective on clinical human suffering. *British Gestalt Journal, 24*(1), 5–19.

Francesetti, G. (2019). A clinical exploration of atmospheres: Towards a field based clinical practice. In G. Francesetti & T. Griffero (Eds.), *Psychopathology and atmospheres: Neither inside nor outside* (p. 35). Cambridge Scholars Publishing.

Freud, S. (1995). *The interpretation of dreams* (A. A. Brill, Trans.). Quality Paperback Book Club. (Original work published 1899)

Grant, A. (2010). Writing the reflexive self: An autoethnography of alcoholism and the impact of psychotherapy culture. *Journal of Psychiatric and Mental Health Nursing, 17*(7), 577–582. https://doi.org/10.1111/j.1365-2850.2010.01566.x

Greenberg, L. S. (1986). Change process research. *Journal of Consulting and Clinical Psychology, 54*(1), 4–9. https://doi.org/10.1037/0022-006X.54.1.4

Jacobs, L., & Hycner, R. (2009). *Relational approaches in Gestalt therapy*. Routledge: Taylor & Francis Group.

Jones, E. E. (2015). Somatic psychotherapy: Illuminating an embodied experience of self-transformation through autoethnography. *Social Work Master's Clinical Research Papers, 461*. https://ir.stthomas.edu/ssw_mstrp/461

Lewin, K. (1951). *Field theory in social science: Selected theoretical papers* (D. Cartwright, Ed.). Harpers.

Lutz, W., Castonguay, L. G., Lambert, M. J., & Barkham, M. (2021). Traditions and new beginnings: Historical and current perspectives on research in psychotherapy and behavior change. In M. Barkham, W. Lutz, & L. G. Castonguay (Eds.), *Bergin and Garfield's handbook of psychotherapy and behavior change* (7th ed., pp. 3–18). John Wiley & Sons.

Moustakas, C. (1990). *Heuristic research. Design, methodology, and applications*. Sage.

Parlett, M. (1991). Reflections on field theory. *The British Gestalt Journal, 1*(1), 69–80.

Perls, F. S. (1992). *Gestalt Therapy Verbatim*. Gestalt Journal Press. (Original work published 1969)

Philippson, P. (2009). *The emergent self. An existential-Gestalt approach*. Karnac Books.

Poulos, C. N. (2021). *Essentials of autoethnography*. APA.

Siddique, S. (2011). Being in-between: The relevance of ethnography and auto-ethnography for psychotherapy research. *Counselling and Psychotherapy Research, 11*(4), 310–316. https://doi.org/10.1080/14733145.2010.533779

Staemmler, F. (2006). A Babylonian confusion? On the uses and meanings of the term 'field'. *British Gestalt Journal, 15*(2), 64.

Talbot, M. (2018). Gestalt psychotherapy, conflict and resolution: An autoethnography. *European Journal for Qualitative Research in Psychotherapy, 8*, 43–53. https://www.ejqrp.org/index.php/ejqrp/article/view/52

Weil, S. (1952). *Gravity and grace* (A. Wills, Trans.). Putnam's Sons.

Yontef, G. M. (1993). *Awareness, dialogue & process: Essays on Gestalt therapy.* (Kindle ed.). The Gestalt Journal Press.

OPEN ACCESS

Being seen: The lived experience of psychodynamic practitioners disclosing or not disclosing sight impairment

Laura Evers

ABSTRACT

The taboo of therapist self-disclosure and literature addressing disclosure and disability issues from a psychodynamic perspective is explored. Research on disclosure decisions among physically impaired practitioners is limited. Interpretative Phenomenological Analysis qualitative research methodology was employed to understand the lived experience of psychodynamic practitioners with sight impairment to understand disclosure decision-making processes in a therapeutic setting. Six participants self-identified as sight impaired psychodynamic practitioners and were interviewed using a semi-structured questionnaire. Findings showed that the experience of working as a practitioner with sight impairment is a tenacious endeavour, requiring high levels of self-awareness and determination in navigating the minefield of self-disclosure, daring to be seen by others, holding the patient's need to be seen and journeying through loss and acceptance of the changing self. Results showed that there is an inverse relationship between likelihood to self-disclose sight impairment and the extent to which practitioners work with unconscious process and transference. Ultimately, the capacity to reclaim disavowed parts of the self, defined therapists' ability to make therapeutic disclosure decisions. Suggestions for future research, clinical and ethical implications are provided plus recommendations for impaired practitioners and those who work with difference.

> We see the things themselves, the world is what we see [. . .] But what is strange about this faith is that if we seek to articulate it into theses or statements, if we ask ourselves what is this *we*, what *seeing* is, and what *thing* and *world* is, we enter into a labyrinth of difficulties and contradictions. (Original italics)
>
> (Merleau-Ponty, 1968 p. 3)

Self-disclosure in its broadest definition is so ubiquitous it is hardly noticed in everyday life. However, for the therapist and especially the therapist who is (in)visibly sight impaired (SI), questions of self-disclosure are considered deeply in terms of conscious and unconscious communication in psychodynamic practice.

Merleau-Ponty (1968) thoughts on the nature of seeing, and Winnicott's (1971) comments on being seen in the 'Mirror-role of Mother' in *Playing and Reality* draw attention to the idea that seeing is a multifaceted process which was considered by Jacobs (1998) in this journal over 20 years ago. Jacobs (1998 p. 214) considers non-verbal communication in the context of seeing and being seen and notes that 'visually impaired therapists or clients may have different experiences from those described below, which . . . would be of great interest to sighted therapists'

Since then, little research was found in the literature that considers the effect of a therapist's sight impairment and how this connects with self-disclosure decisions. The desire to respond to Jacobs' expression of interest initiated the question for this research.

The experience under investigation is how 'being seen' is altered when the therapist's sight is impaired and observation skills are conceptualised differently. In these circumstances, non-verbal and verbal communication, including self-disclosures are taking place as in any therapeutic relationship (Hobson, 1989). The question that emerges is how do therapists with sight impairment decide whether to verbally disclose their (dis)ability – whether it can be seen or remains unseen by the client – and how is this experienced consciously and unconsciously by therapist and client from the therapist's perspective?

The origin of the question and research aims

While there is guidance written by able-bodied therapists for counselling impaired clients (Segal, 1996, 2006; Wilson, 2003, 2006), literature for therapists who are impaired is scarce (White, 2011). Qualitative research involving participants with SI is sparse (Barr et al., 2012; Groneck, 2013; Thurston, 2010). *The British Journal of Visual Impairment, Journal of Visual Impairment and Blindness*, and *Disability and Society* have some contributors who consider issues of counselling people with SI and the experience of being sight impaired and some of those contributors disclose their own visual or other impairments (e.g. French, 1995; Shakespeare, 1994; Thurston, 2010; Thurston et al., 2013). Within psychotherapy literature, the quiet voice of therapists with impairments may reflect a broader phenomenon, conceptualised by Shakespeare (1994) as 'invasion':

> It is not only physical limitations that restrict us to our homes and those whom we know. It is the knowledge that each entry into the public world will be dominated by stares, by condescension, by pity and by hostility.
>
> (*Shakespeare.*, p. 288, quoting Morris)

The temptation, with non-obvious SI, is to 'get away with it' (Phillips, 2012) and not to be seen as impaired by others, a 'disavowal' of absence of sight (Freud, 1940) or 'superblind', as the SI community describe people with SI who function as if sighted (Borg, 2005). 'Coming out' (Kleege, 1999; O'Connell, 2011) is a disclosure that creates a tension against getting away with it. Is it necessary to say anything at all? What about remaining 'neutral' (Jacobs, 2004)? Would it ever be noticeable, and if no one said anything did that mean they hadn't noticed, or did they notice and say nothing? Are clients unconsciously aware of everything anyway (Joseph, 1985)? Would disclosure or non-disclosure 'disable' the process (Segal, 1996)? Therapists in clinical practice find themselves precariously balanced on the threshold between being seen and not being seen. This liminal place is potentially a place of creativity, and is also defined by frustration and not knowing. Kuusisto (1998, pp. 11–12) conceptualises this as being in the customs house 'between the ocean of blindness and the land of seeing [...] It's a transitory place, its foundation shifting, its promise of stasis always suspect'.

This research seeks the assistance of visually impaired practitioners in thinking about the nature of seeing and being seen. Its purpose is to add to the literature on managing disclosure of therapist impairment in the counselling room. The hope is that something can be added to the debate on disclosure and impairment and that it might have wider implications for considering therapist illness, aging and other challenges to therapists' perceptions of themselves as able.

This research aims to investigate two main aspects of therapist self -disclosure (TSD); the intersubjective process of how, why, when and what therapists decide to disclose to clients and in what circumstances, and how therapists disclose to themselves in order to engage in the intrasubjective process of therapeutic gain.

Literature review

A search of literature revealed no existing empirical or theoretical literature specifically exploring all elements of this research: *TSD* issues among *psychodynamic practitioners* with *SI in the UK*. Some studies partially explore these elements (Axelman & Kashani, 2009; Bottrill et al., 2009; Burke Valeras, 2007; Calonico, 1995; Carew, 2009; Hansen, 2008; Hernandez, 2011; Jeffery & Tweed, 2014; Mallinckrodt & Helms, 1986; Moore & Jenkins, 2012; O'Connell, 2011; Parker, 2011; Pizer, 2016; Shapiro, 1990; Stanley et al., 2011).

The starting point was the literature on self-disclosure and non-disclosure leading to the literature on disability and impairment in general. These two areas are then drawn together by reviewing the small body of literature which combines TSD and impairment.

Theoretical orientation and TSD: The debate for and against TSD

The debate about TSD is marked by controversy resulting in a dichotomized views based on theoretical schools of thought, cultural context, definitions and therapeutic effects (Wachtel, 2011). One aspect that doesn't provoke conflict is the complexity and ill-defined nature of TSD. Bloomgarden and Mennuti (2009), Farber (2006), Henretty and Levitt (2010), Maroda (2010), Peterson (2002) and Stricker and Fisher (1990) are agreed that every therapist needs to reflect on their interventions and navigate the question of self-disclosure, based on their own circumstances, individual relationships with each client and with the interests of the client at the centre. Henretty and Levitt (2010) point out, in their extensive qualitative review of over 30 predominately North American research studies, that 90% of therapists self-disclose at some point. However, TSD represents only 3.5% of all therapist interventions suggesting TSD is used by many but sparingly. Despite the vast body of research conducted, Henretty and Levitt (2010 p. 64) conclude therapists are left feeling vulnerable and anxious about TSD because of ambiguity and contradictions in training, ethical guidelines, empirical findings and theoretical conceptualizations.

Pro-disclosure perspective

Sydney Jourard is credited with the first use of the term 'self-disclosure' when in 1964 he assessed people's likelihood to disclose aspects of themselves to others (Cozby, 1973 p.73). In the 1950s, Rogerians were the first clinicians to adopt TSD in practice (Farber, 2006). Those from a humanistic tradition used TSD to communicate congruence, positive regard, authenticity, transparency and equalise the balance of power in the therapeutic relationship. Since then, client-centred therapists have argued that by cautiously modelling openness, strength, vulnerability and sharing intense feelings, the therapist invites the client to follow their lead. The outcome intended is the creation of trust though perceived similarity, credibility and empathic understanding (Bloomgarden & Mennuti, 2009; Henretty & Levitt, 2010). Segal (1993 p. 13), who writes from a Kleinian perspective, also emphasises the importance of being client-centred but without necessarily modelling via TSD: "being 'client-centred' doesn't mean doing everything the client wants you to do".

Non-disclosure perspective

Though critics accuse Freud of breaking his own rules on anonymity, neutrality and abstinence (Lane & Hull, 1990), many of these infringements occurred during the early years of the development of psychoanalysis

(Farber, 2006; Peterson, 2002). What remains in psychoanalytic tradition is the idea of remaining a neutral and anonymous medium, upon which patients can project transference distortions for the purpose of interpretation (Farber, 2006).

Freud's comment on technique (Freud, 1912 p. 111) suggests the oft-cited use of 'evenly-suspended attention' and posture of the analyst as: 'opaque to his patients and, like a mirror, should show them nothing but what is shown to him' (Freud, 1912 p. 118). Less often quoted is what Freud writes next, that in practice 'some suggestive influence', which could be seen as Freud's term for TSD, may be combined with analysis 'in order to gain a perceptible result in a shorter time – as is necessary for instance, in institutions' (Freud, 1912 p. 118). Freud concedes this is a valid method but cannot be called true psychoanalysis in his terms. A contemporary proponent of this is Coren (2010, p. 162) who suggests that in short-term work, TSD can be effective in building alliance and short-circuiting clients' defences.

It is on Freud's definition of true psychoanalysis that perhaps the debate on self-disclosure seems to hang. Many quote Freud's idea that disclosure begets disclosure. Jourard (1971), for example, implies that client disclosure is the goal in and of itself. Freud (1912 p. 118) suggests the patient may feel obliged to reciprocate with a confidence they are already aware of. The psychoanalytic aim is to discover what lies in the unconscious and cannot be accessed so readily. The focus on the unconscious is a 'principle hypothesis of psychodynamic work' (Jacobs, 2004 p. 11) and central to the debate about TSD. Examples of contemporary thinkers in line with Freud's focus on the unconscious, and therefore on the non-disclosing end of the disclosure spectrum, include Langs (1998), Lemma (2003) and Segal (1993). Maroda (2010) and Bridges (2001) integrate some of the differences outlined above.

Contemporary thinking on TSD is summarised by Billow (2000 p. 66) after an extensive review of literature prior to 2000: 'the rule is there are no hard and fast rules. One guideline is to consider whether they [TSD] work to open or close things up between patient and analyst'. The question is not whether to disclose or not but to reflect on how TSD affects the therapeutic process.

The literature suggests the decision to disclose to a client is a nuanced, non-binary decision dependent on theoretical orientation and differing perceptions of *how* client needs are met.

Impairment and sight impairment

Wilson (2003 p. 12) suggests that the relative absence of psychoanalytic writing about disability and death anxiety suggests a link between the two and recommends that to work with disability requires resolution of death anxiety and awareness of defences, especially that of denial. A search of the

Psychodynamic Practice and *Counselling* and *Psychotherapy Research* journals confirmed that since Wilson's (2003) comment, there is only a small body of literature in UK publications in the area of impairment and SI (Barr et al., 2012; Charmaz, 1995; Fitzerman, 1996; Segal, 1996; Spencer, 2000; Thurston, 2010; Thurston et al., 2013; Wilson, 2003, 2006).

The broad messages from the review are: 1) psychoanalytic theory is useful in constructing a model for thinking about impairment because it articulates integration of the individual's internal and external world with society; 2) the role of 'others' (supervisors/employees) in the lives of therapists with impairments is critical in defining their experience of being impaired and working therapeutically.

Models of disability

Models of disability are constructs that frame thinking about disability and are a common starting point for many writers in Clinical Psychology, Sociology and Psychotherapy (Bickenbach et al., 1999; Fitzerman, 1996; Goodley, 2011; Olkin, 2002; O'Connell, 2011; Shakespeare & Watson, 2002; Watermeyer, 2012; Wilson, 2003). The medical, moral and society models conceptualize the differing ways in which others have viewed people with a disability (Olkin, 2002). Shakespeare (1994), Goodley (2011) and Watermeyer (2012) make a case for the value of psychoanalytic thought in the society model by drawing together the role of society and the individual. Watermeyer (2012 p. 171) cites Fanon's concept of internalised oppression to suggest that a disabled person's unconscious collusion with societal discrimination against the disabled body as an out-group will result in a 'recapitulation of the status quo'. Watermeyer advocates for consciously processing these traumatic internalisations therapeutically.

Psychodynamics and impairment

Asch and Rousso (1985) and Cubbage and Thomas (1989) provide an overview of the relevance of Freud's work for disability, argung for the inclusion of therapists with impairments in psychotherapeutic practice. Grzesiak and Hicok (1994 p. 249) offer a brief history of psychotherapy and physical disability suggesting that there are no differences in working with those who have physical difficulties than with "so-called 'ordinary people'". They outline relevant areas of psychodynamic theory for impairment; mourning and loss, secondary gain, trauma, ego defences, castration anxiety and narcissistic injury. Wilson (2003) reviews different psychodynamic approaches to working with impairment.

Goffman (1963) is a Canadian sociologist referred to by many writers (Burke Valeras, 2007; Fitzerman, 1996; French, 1995; Hernandez, 2011;

O'Connell, 2011; Vick, 2007). His seminal text on stigma and the ideas of 'covering' and 'passing' are made contemporary by Yoshino (2007 p. ix). To 'cover' is to tone down a disfavoured identity to fit into the mainstream; to choose not to be known as different. 'passing' is to adopt a 'don't ask don't tell' attitude, where difference is known but ignored. While these are not psychodynamic theoretical ideas, they connect with the theory on disavowal (Freud, 1940) and provide routes into thinking dynamically about the stigma often associated with impairment.

Winnicott's (1971) elaborates on Lacan's concept of the mirror phase, as a reflection of a child's emerging self; a reflection of the baby in the mother's eyes.

> When I look I am seen, so I exist.
> I can now afford to look and see.
> I now look creatively and what I appreciate I also perceive.
> In fact I take care not to see what is not there to be seen (unless I am tired)
>
> (Winnicott, 1971 p. 134)

In this paradoxical riddle, the notion of 'being seen' in the psychological sense is linked to the literal ability of the mother to see (Jacobs, 1998). An implicit fear of remaining unseen is the atrophy of creative capacity and a failure to find oneself reflected back by the environment (Winnicott, 1971 p. 131). Winnicott's (1971) draws attention to the idea that a mother will find other sensory ways of communicating her recognition of the baby if the baby is blind but doesn't consider the effect of a care giver's SI.

Issues of loss of body unity and loss of omnipotent feelings are associated with impairment. Charmaz (1995, p. 357) suggests adapting to impairment means 'struggling with rather than against illness'. Chernin (1976) reflects that when he acknowledged his own omnipotent feelings, he could also accept his illness and limitations which released him from the guilt of leaving his patients in need.

Fitzerman (1996) was the only author found who self-discloses a visible physical impairment and writes from a psychodynamic perspective. She suggests that anger is likely to be present, even if not acknowledged by an impaired client, and is a defence against depression and narcissistic injury. While acknowledging her impairment, the focus of her article is on clients not therapists with impairments.

TSD and impairment research

Miller (1991 p. 348) reviews the literature before 1991 and considers both additive and subtractive points of view found in research assessing client response to therapist impairment. Miller suggests that therapists self-disclosing a disability at the beginning stage of the counselling process are 'probably safe to do so'. O'Connell (2011) researches TSD of therapists with visible physical disabilities and concludes that disclosure of disability-related material should be initiated by the therapist early in the therapeutic encounter and be phrased in an open-ended way that leaves room for future discussion (O'Connell, 2011 p. 74).

Methodology

Interpretative Phenomenological Analysis (IPA) was chosen as disability and impairment are phenomena that are often generalised and individual experience is lost. This research adopts an ideographic qualitative approach because 'no two people experience disability in the same way, just as no two people experience life in the same way' (Wilson, 2003 p. ix).

The research inhabits 'insider' status (Smith et al., 2009 p. 42) describing the researcher's eye condition in the recruitment letter for transparency when asking participants to discuss their eyesight in the research. By disclosing, the dynamic was set for the interview in a research frame, providing participants with the freedom to respond without the special conditions of a therapist-client dyad. Every effort was made to bracket the researcher's response and experience as a therapist with SI, but it is inevitable that unconscious aspects of the researcher's fore-concepts (Finlay, 1999) influence this work.

Ethical approval was received and participants were recruited by referral and through snowballing (Smith et al., 2009). Due to the nature of the research, careful consideration was given to accessibility and this was managed on a case-by-case basis according to the participants' needs. Six, sixty minute interviews were conducted with psychodynamic practitioners with at least one year's post qualification experience. All research participants self-identified as having SI, which might suggest a degree of similarity in the way that participants experienced 'seeing'. However, each participant had an individual experience of sight loss and of working with SI. The physical eye conditions were described as: Lattice Dystrophy and Horner's syndrome, Glaucoma, Sjogrens Syndrome, Retinopathy of Prematurity, Retinitis Pigmentosa, Retinopathy with Glaucoma and total blindness (cause not specified).

Co-created researcher/participant vignettes enable each individual's circumstances to be known (names have been changed for anonymity)

Mary is 61, qualified as an integrative counsellor 16 years ago and works in student counselling and private practice. Her experience of sight change began as she was training. She has a fluctuating condition, which can change quickly, sometimes hour-to-hour, reducing access to sight significantly. When needed, Mary uses magnification devices and wears dark glasses.

Hazel is mid to late 50s. She has 30 years' experience working as a psychodynamic counsellor and 14 years as a psychoanalytic psychotherapist in both education and medical sectors. Hazel lost 95% of her sight as a young adult and the remaining 5% six years ago. Her guide dog is present in her room for therapeutic sessions, unless clients ask for it to be removed. She uses a symbol cane and computer software, which translates written text to speech.

Georgia is in her mid 60s. She initially trained psychodynamically but now identifies herself as integrative, having additionally studied Play Therapy, Gestalt and Transactional Analysis. She is experienced in telephone and online counselling and has her own private practice. Georgia has two eye conditions: one, diagnosed 20 years ago, is degenerative but doesn't influence the way she practices as yet, and the other, recently diagnosed (three years ago), results in eye watering/dryness. She manages her eye condition with eye drops which lubricate and reduce irritation. She also wears tinted and photochromic glasses to reduce the effects of light conditions. Georgia uses magnification devices for reading

Amanda is 53 and qualified as a psychodynamic counsellor two years ago. She works in private practice and for a health organisation. Amanda's experience of sight change began 14 years ago. She has a fluctuating condition which can change quickly, reducing access to sight significantly. Her sight is currently better than it has been. Amanda uses magnification devices and a white stick when travelling. In the therapeutic setting she sometimes wears glasses with one frosted lens.

Elizabeth is in her early 70s and has been practising as a psychoanalyst for 30 years. She offers long-term analysis in private practice. Elizabeth's eye condition has been evident for many years but developed life-changing consequences in 1988 when she stopped driving. It is a degenerative condition, resulting in a narrowed field of vision. She uses a white stick outside and is about to acquire a guide dog.

Steve is 63, qualified as a counsellor 12 years ago and works short- and long-term with couples and individuals. Steve was born unsighted but could perceive light/dark until a haemorrhage in his eyes as a young adult caused complete sight loss. Steve uses a Braille Notetaker in assessments as his pen and paper. When he had a guide dog, he didn't take it into therapeutic sessions to avoid possible distraction.

Research results

Phenomenological themes

'Tenacious endeavour' defines the essential quality of all six participants' experience of working as therapists with SI. Three master themes demonstrate how the phenomenon of 'Tenacious endeavour' is experienced in the therapeutic setting, in the world with others and internally.

(i) Navigating complexity in the minefield of TSD: investigates the experience of engaging in the therapeutic process.

> 'Self-disclosure, . . . is a real minefield. I would go very warily along that route'.

(ii) Standing firm under fire: explores the experience of working with others, clients' and authority figures' projections and prejudice.

> 'I had (hesitating tone) major battles, in that the issue of disclosure came up . . . it was thought that my patients should be informed in advance that I was blind'.

(iii) The journey from loss to acceptance: considers the experience of the changing self.

> 'When I got the first diagnosis, . . . it was quite a shock . . . I ran a thing about; "will I be blind within a year?" Calmed down . . . and had some extra therapy'

Nuanced and complex sub-themes emerged within master themes and they are reflected in the framework for results in Figure 1.

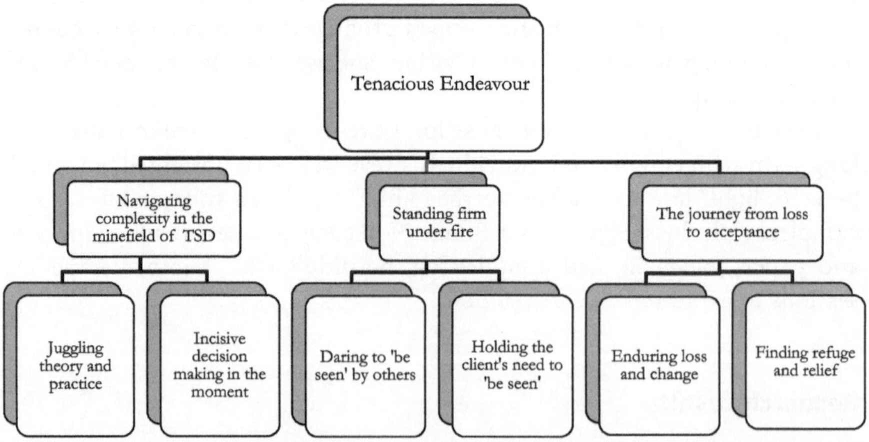

Figure 1. Framework for results.

Juggling theory and practice

Every participant discussed their approach to self-disclosure with reference to their training and theoretical model in terms that either distanced them from or kept them close to their original psychodynamic training. Each participant juggled theory and practice in different ways.

The sense of juggling comes from three elements that seemed to be perpetually in motion and sometimes in tension:

(i) Implementing training and theoretical models in practice.
(ii) Assessing potential and unknown therapeutic outcomes of TSD.
(iii) Building the therapeutic relationship.

In order to conceptualise the different approaches to juggling these three elements, participants' approaches are located on a spectrum from non-disclosure to pro-disclosure as: classic (non-disclosure), experimental and non-conformist (pro-disclosure).

Classic approach: Hazel and Elizabeth took the most faithful approach to classic psychodynamic theory with regard to TSDSI in inhabiting a predominately non-disclosing position. Non-verbal disclosures are acknowledged as inevitable and SI is grouped with all other non-verbal/factual disclosures. For Hazel, TSDSI is used therapeutically in the context of managing transference distortions. For example:

> You can represent the impaired parent ... I do have real empathy for [the client], if there's been a sibling ... or a parent whose been disabled. I'm very mindful that the transference can be *very* (emphasis) powerful ... and possibly too powerful for the person ... to tolerate.

In these circumstances, TSDSI is used to elevate painful and potentially unhelpful transference.

Experimental approach: Amanda and Mary were experimental in their approach to TSDSI, trying things out and then modifying their approach based on their eye conditions' fluctuations and their experience with clients.

Amanda acknowledged that non-verbal disclosure makes a totally purist approach impossible. 'I'm not a tabula rasa' and experimented with factual TSDSI in the first session. Amanda acknowledges that 'there are arguments about this and I'm not sure that there's a right or wrong approach'. A client with cerebral palsy responded silently to first session TSDSI and changed the subject, but did not return. Amanda felt she had 'made a mistake' by taking something away from the client in disclosing SI:

> I set up competition ... she wasn't coping very well and here was I, in her phantasy of me, I was okay, then I told her that I've got this disability

Based on experience, Amanda has shifted to a position where she waits for a natural moment to disclose her sight condition.

Non-conformist approach: Georgia and Steve, though starting with training that promoted non-disclosure, have moved to pro-disclosure positions. Georgia uses experience in her own therapy to develop her stance on TSD:

> It's the human edge where therapy works. I'm not just going to . . . behave like an automaton, I've experienced a few of those . . . it's like there are certain religions . . . if you're not with us you're *dammed* (emphasis) forever and I think I'm one of the eternal "don't knows", . . . It's their therapy not mine (pause) which is why when I'm in therapy I wanted it to be my therapy (sigh)

The need for therapeutic alliance takes precedence over the classical non-disclosing stance. However, Georgia was less pro-TSDSI, especially if SI is less obvious. At whatever point on the spectrum therapists were located, all were agreed on the importance of decisions being made for client benefit.

Incisive decision making in the moment

All participants were clear that TSDSI decisions were made on an individual basis and were dependent on client presentation and therapeutic goals. For example, Elizabeth commented that she wouldn't use TSDSI with a borderline patient. Mary said she was less likely to use TSDSI with a short-term client. It was evident from the data that therapists thought deeply about when and why they would use TSDSI, as summarised by Elizabeth:

> I don't know whether I'd say, . . . 'I don't see things', and I may say that meaning, I don't see things literally or I don't see things in a psychological sense, I'm not understanding something, and that the two would be concomitant really. Which I would take up, I can't say categorically because I'd be playing it by ear.

Although participants had differing views, there was agreement that the timing of effective TSDSI is critical. This demonstrates the skill of holding back on opportunities for disclosure, in pursuit of precise and well-timed interventions necessary to make effective TSDSI for therapeutic gain.

Daring to 'be seen' by others

While taking a stand with colleagues and organisations invoked rage at the unnecessary nature of such battles, there was a willingness to stand firm against the hostile projections of others, in order to hold their need to 'be seen' as part of the therapeutic process using TSD where necessary.

All participants commented on times when they had been forced into a position of having to take a stand with a training organisation or employer/colleague in order to defend their ability or needs.

Hazel had 'major battles' with the training organisation's policy of disclosing her blindness pre-first session:

> I was really discouraged from challenging it [by supervisor], the feeling was that I would actually put my training at risk. I was told 'don't rock the boat'

Hazel felt individuals acted out prejudice in the organisation. She was successful on her own behalf but didn't change policy for those who followed. Incidents of conflict have long-lasting effects on the internal world of those with impairments as acknowledged by Hazel at the end of the interview:

> I think what I've realised is, that whole training experience still has raw edges, that really pissed me off (low voice).

Talking about the experience of 14 years ago activated rage still deeply felt and suggests that daring to be seen as impaired is costly but essential to gain access to professional therapeutic training.

Steve describes himself as a therapist who is blind rather than a blind therapist. He adapted this language to communicate his ability despite what others, his past employers in this case, might perceive as a disability.

> I was aware that as a blind person you had to fight to get what you believed you could do . . . I didn't want to appear as someone who had a chip on their shoulder but on the other hand I wanted to stand my ground if I believed in it.

Mary had the experience of being treated like everyone else when she needed to be treated differently. Personal printers were removed in favour of communal ones, making access to printed information complex:

> it's [SI] acknowledged at appraisals. . . it's just when resources get squeezed everybody gets squeezed regardless, ...it's so trivial but, . . . it can't be understood can it really, how it affects us and what it means for us in terms of our life

Although Mary stood her ground and got through the necessary 'red tape', she was left with feeling unnoticed and misunderstood.

Holding clients' need to 'be seen'

There were rich examples of how therapists hold clients without seeing. The few represented here show both the creativity and challenge that therapists engage with in the task of holding the client.

All participants demonstrated ways in which they had adapted to SI and observed the client without seeing them, holding their clients' need to be seen:

> You can hear it in the voice ... You can pick up when somebody is not making eye contact with you because the voice shifts .... You can hear the tears .... You can sense that they're tucked into a corner or sitting on the edges of the seat

Amanda refers to her use of countertransference as a tool for observing:

> I've always been very alert to countertransference, but I think this [SI] is another dimension to it that I'm aware of, and picking up on unconscious processes ... may or may not be to do with [SI], but just the fact that there might be makes me tune in more.

All participants talked about the difficulty of dealing with client projections, the fear of death, association with vulnerability and loss that can be evoked by proximity to impairment:

> I've had to deal with the *hostility* towards me because I'm blind or shall I say hostility towards me which got expressed around my blindness.

Hazel made sense of the experience of this hostility by outlining her view on where the hostility was coming from, summarized here as:

(i) People are terrified that they too could lose their sight and a lot of the hostility is a projection of that fear.
(ii) They project their own vulnerability onto me, if they don't want to face that vulnerability themselves; they want to get rid of me and thereby get rid of it.
(iii) I think it's sometimes envy and attempting to spoil what I have.

Enduring loss and change

The journey from loss to acceptance is divided into two sub-themes: 'enduring loss and change', which considers therapists' experience of coming to terms with the changing self; and 'finding refuge and relief', which outlines the places where therapists find relief from isolation.

Five participants talked about enduring ongoing losses that occurred after initial diagnosis. Georgia recognised the process of coming to terms with SI as a series of losses not a one-off experience:

> it's not just about the disability is it? It's about how psychologically we deal with it, which can be very erratic. It's not like you get the diagnosis and then you have the breakdown. It's several years later you suddenly get that jerk which is 'ooh my last test wasn't as good.

For those with fluctuating conditions (three participants) the sight loss process was unpredictable and sometimes unbearable; the future is unknown and frightening:

> The disease eats into the corneas . . . it's unbearable, so I've had two grafts on the left eye, but they weren't successful . . . didn't get the vision back. So I just fear for the right eye when the time comes . . . . Err, (pause) that I won't get vision back.

Five participants acknowledged the difficulty of enduring sight loss and could identify in themselves tendencies for disavowal, 'Part of me wants to disavow the whole thing. I have to admit to that really'. There was a strong desire not to be noticed as different, 'not to be seen to be vulnerable . . . . not to be seen to be out of the ordinary. Um, (slight pause) I'm getting less inhibited'.

The fear of being seen to be vulnerable was based on associations that were hard to own, 'I don't know whether you call it pride or a wish to be in a position of strength . . . when I articulate it, it sounds stupid in a way'.

The process of accepting the changing self requires in-depth reflection. Amanda found therapy a helpful place to process her changing sight, identity as a therapist and attitudes to TSDSI:

> I made the decision that I wasn't going to disclose because of how it was making me feel about my own sight loss . . . I think this is quite important to say, that I was almost apologizing for it.

Finding refuge and relief

Identifying places where therapists seek refuge and relief was not part of the question structure, but five participants mentioned at least one experience where they had found refuge and relief from the loneliness of facing the challenges of SI.

Therapists and supervisors were most often referred to as a place of refuge:

> If somebody else can understand. I mean it's just not something you want to talk about, or other people want to talk about is it? It's good to talk to my supervisor, . . . to have an outlet of frustration and how it does affect me.

Clinical and theoretical implications

The aims of this research were to explore the lived experience of psychodynamic practitioners with SI and to understand their approach to TSDSI. The main finding runs implicitly throughout all result sections but is most evident in the phenomenon of 'juggling theory and practice'. The research found that there is an inverse relationship between likelihood to use TSDSI and the extent to which practitioners work with unconscious process and transference. This is consistent with Carew's (2009) findings. Participants who work with the 'classic approach' tend to use TSDSI, only when relevant to transference and interpretation of unconscious communication, avoiding first session disclosure. The 'non-conformist approach' led participants to focus more on the therapeutic alliance and 'being human'. TSD was used to facilitate the process of open communication especially in the early stages of therapeutic relationship development.

Three main factors are considered in making decisions about TSDSI:

(i) How does TSDSI affect development of transference?
(ii) How will TSDSI contribute to building the therapeutic alliance?
(iii) What are the likely outcomes of TSDSI in relation to therapeutic goals?

Practitioners make TSDSI decisions by using a combination of their training and theoretical positions, experiences of working with SI, in-depth reflection and monitoring of the changing self. TSDSI decisions are tailored to the client's unique circumstances and the intersubjectivity of each therapeutic dyad. The experience of sustaining this level of diligence in addition to the ordinary challenges of being a psychodynamic practitioner is interpreted phenomenologically as a tenacious endeavour.

Issues that drive the decision-making process for TSDSI are the client's impairment stability and noticeability, the extent of client disturbance and type of disturbance, the therapist's approach to transference and unconscious process and the likely therapeutic gain of TSDSI.

The nature of seeing and being seen

This research found that the notion of noticeability is a subjective construct in line with Merleau-Ponty's (1968) philosophy. Client observation skills are variable, determined by the client's eyesight, preoccupation with his or her own concerns and natural observations skills. Therapist's with SI grapple with how seen a client is in a literal sense, and how 'seen' the client feels, in the psychological sense. Participants spoke about times when clients had been unable to tolerate being unseen, in both versions of the meaning of 'being seen' and could also give examples of what a relief it might be for clients not to 'be seen'. The results provided evidence that therapists endeavour to ensure that they are self-aware and reflective on a client-by-client basis and are creative and dedicated to the work of holding their clients' need to 'be seen'.

If literal seeing and psychological understanding become concomitant, Winnicott's (1971) notion of the primitive fear of not being seen can become activated. Underpinning any other therapeutic goals, the therapist with SI must embrace the association between the unseen and the need to be seen. For clients, It could be therapeutic to overcome primitive fear and recognise that it is possible to be seen psychologically without being seen literally.

When the therapist is sight-impaired this is part of the work, either consciously via disclosure or through unconscious communication.

The results showed that disavowal is, at varying degrees of conscious recognition, an issue with which therapists must engage. Disavowal (Britton, 1994; Fitzerman, 1996; Shakespeare, 1994) is a defence that needs special consideration on the part of the therapists with SI. The results show that therapists with SI endeavour to unearth the areas that could 'disable' the therapeutic process, and engage with the desire to deny difficulty and avoid the issues raised by absent or limited sight (Segal, 1996). Some participants experienced a unique difficulty working with impaired clients consistent with Fitzerman's (1996) and Borg's (2005) observations of working with impaired clients who may feel competition and envy towards the impaired therapist.

Participants' experience of 'being seen by others' were in line with Goodley's (2011) and Watermeyer's (2012) papers on the connection between societal oppression and internal oppression. Society's impact on individual experience of the self as impaired can be disabling. Participants articulated ways in which they had 'been seen' by others in both helpful and less helpful ways. To varying degrees, participants acknowledged that the ability to 'stand firm' requires awareness of the need to resist introjected forms of society's oppression. Participants' experiences of 'standing firm' resonated with those of Kleege (1999), Kuusisto (1998) and Yoshino (2007) and echoed themes of 'getting away with it' (Phillips, 2012), 'covering/passing' (Goffman, 1963) and 'coming out' (O'Connell, 2011).

Ethical aspects of working as a therapist with sight impairment

The results showed that participants struggled to self-disclose their disability to colleagues in organizations because of past negative experiences. Places where participants expected to find refuge and relief were sometimes places of difficulty and required tenacious endeavour to gain access to what they needed, exemplified by Mary's printer battle and Hazel's fight for training patients. In training organisations and employment settings, able-bodied individuals act out organisational, societal and personal defences against engaging with impairment which disable the therapist with SI. This forced participants to stand their ground and seek other places of refuge and relief with family, supervisors or therapists who can understand the traumatising nature of these experiences.

There is a difference between having a good disability policy in place and acting in the spirit of those policies in everyday life (Olkin, 2002). It seemed that it was in the every day 'trivial(Mary)' details of being trained or working that therapists with SI experienced difficulty and discrimination, which detracted from the primary task of working therapeutically with clients.

The BACP ethical guidelines (Bond et al., 2013) state that 'practitioners should not allow their professional relationships with colleagues to be prejudiced by their own personal views about a colleague's [. . .] disability' (Bond et al., 2013 p. 9). It is easy to agree with this on paper, while the experience of not allowing prejudice to encroach on the day-to-day lives of practitioners with impairments seems difficult to navigate. The logical corollary to this is how a therapist with impaired sight can respond to these 'trivial' yet prejudiced experiences. This will be considered in recommendations for practice.

While the research did not specifically focus on ethical guidelines and how participants thought about 'fitness to practice', it was evident from the interviews that practitioners considered their ability to work and continually monitored themselves in supervision.

Participants reported a mixed experience of working with supervisors ranging from a great level of comfort in discussing issues relevant to SI to a degree of discomfort. The supervisor's ability to work with difference in terms of willingness and skill were central to participants' experience in supervision. This is consistent with Spencer's (2000) thoughts on the need to develop potential space and provide proactive support.

Lifecycles of becoming

The phenomenon of 'enduring loss and change' attempts to capture the sense of the loss that endures over a long period and also bearing the weight of significant loss and change. Implicit in the research findings is the connection between the experience of becoming impaired and becoming a therapist. It has been argued that both processes involve coming to terms with loss; loss of a former self (Charmaz, 1995) or the loss of omnipotent feelings (Chernin, 1976). The experience of becoming sight-impaired before training (three participants) is a different experience to becoming qualified to practice first and then losing sight (two participants). There is a third experience where becoming a therapist converges with sight loss: only one participant represents this position. The adaption process for those who lose sight after becoming a therapist seems most challenging in TSDSI terms, as there is an accustomed way of working that needs to be adapted and integrated with the changing self. For those who trained as sight-impaired, SI had been integrated into the training process and a professional stance on TSDSI developed, based on an already changed self.

The results confirmed Wilson's (2006) comment on the sense that people with impairments must continually process the difference between Merleau-Ponty's concept of the perfect 'wished for body' and the reality of the 'body in the moment' (Wilson, 2006 p. 178). Inhabiting the space between the wished for and real body creates a sense of being in 'eternal transition'. Participants were at different stages in the process of negotiating the tension between these two bodies. The experience of this tension felt more active among those with fluctuating or degenerative conditions, where TSDSI decisions were continually navigated in day-to-day issues of the working lives of therapists with SI. While those with stable SI did not experience less difficulty, there was a sense of knowing what the difficulty would be each day, as they trained without sight and had been without sight for a long time.

Implications for practice and theory

The need to remain reflective and self-aware was strongly communicated by participants. The necessity of engaging in personal therapy if SI changes or develops for the first time when qualified is key to remaining fit to practice. Recognising potential areas of disavowal and processes of physical loss seem essential for practitioners to consider. An awareness of symbolism and the different ways in which clients may respond to SI given their history and experience is critical to remaining client-centred. The connection between SI and primitive fears of not being seen, feelings of omnipotence, anger and death anxiety are inevitably active in therapeutic work and need to be worked through in order to continue to provide effective therapy for clients.

Being unapologetic for impairment (Chernin, 1976) and embracing adaptation to the changing self (Charmaz, 1995) are important processes, as exemplified explicitly by Amanda who used personal therapy to become unapologetic and changed TSDSI practice in line with that internal shift. This echoes the writing of Watermeyer's (2012) who highlights the benefit of consciously working through unconsciously internalised oppression.

TSDSI decisions need to be weighed against therapeutic goals and the unique needs of each client. The therapist's training and practice will determine how and when TSDSI are made, and while they are always made with the clients' best interests at heart, the therapist's view on beneficence will depend in part of their theoretical stance.

The degree of SI noticeability can affect the decision to disclose with a tendency towards increased use of TSDSI, the more noticeable the impairment. However, when noticeable, some therapists still decide not to self-disclose and wait for the material to lead them. Great attention needs to be paid to the material which clients present and SI is an additional layer that needs to be sought in the material.

Supervisors and therapists of sight-impaired practitioners need to equip themselves with knowledge and understanding of outcomes and issues for practice in order to proactively offer support for those with sight conditions, as underlined by Fitzerman (1996) and Spencer (2000), and in order to prevent their therapeutic relationships with impaired clients or supervisees becoming 'disabled' (Segal, 1996).

Supervisor training on difference could include more detailed research-based findings on working with impairment and specifically how to work through ethical issues of fitness to practice, with guidance on how to translate the principle of working without prejudice into the day-to-day trivial matters that cause therapists with SI to be misunderstood. The provision of reflective space within organisations could create an environment for inevitable issues of prejudice to be worked through in a group. If defences are predicted and thought through in an open, thinking team, client work is less likely to be contaminated by unresolved organisational dynamics.

Ethical guidelines with regard to fitness to practice are open to interpretation. The divergent experiences of therapists with SI in supervision suggest it would be interesting to research these issues at a deeper level, as the definition for 'impairment' in the BACP guidelines seems vague and perhaps deliberately so, giving practitioners the space to navigate this definition for themselves. How to equip practitioners to do this ethical thinking seems lacking in the available literature and initial training.

Olkin (2002) highlights accessibility failures in training. 'We are not training non-disabled psychologists to work with clients with disabilities, nor are we training many psychologists with disabilities. No wonder disabilities have been called the hidden minority' (Olkin, 2002 p. 132). Training courses need to better equip therapists in general and impaired therapists on the issues, debates and conditions where disablism thrives and offer strategies for avoiding them. This may mean looking outside the psychotherapeutic literature and theory as it is currently an underdeveloped area in psychodynamic theory.

Recommendations for further research

Future research could consider taking a 'case study approach' (Smith et al., 2009 p. 52) to more deeply understand the lived experience of psychodynamic therapists' disclosing and living with SI.

The use of a 'triangulation approach' (Smith et al., 2009 p. 53) would also be interesting to gain perspectives of impairment from the point of view of the client, therapist and/or supervisor or organisational representative. Such a study could investigate at deeper levels how difference and impairment were experienced from different perspectives and could include an analysis of how ethical guidelines are worked out in practice.

Ultimately this research concludes that an internal identity shift is needed to re-internalise disavowed parts. Being sight-impaired is to be 'bi-abled' like bi-cultural, an experience of living in two worlds able to adapt one's identity to fit the situation and context (Burke Valeras, 2007 p. 54). Integrating the unable and able parts of the body and mind, known and unknown, in both those who identify as able bodied and as disabled, makes space for therapeutic client-focussed self-disclosure decisions.

Disclosure statement

No potential conflict of interest was reported by the author.

References

Asch, A., & Rousso, H. (1985). Therapists with disabilities: Theoretical and clinical issues. *Psychiatry*, *48*(1), 1–12. https://doi.org/10.1080/00332747.1985.11024263

Axelman, M., & Kashani, D. R. (2009). Issues faced by therapists with visible disabilities: The role of transference, anxiety, and the notion of otherness in the therapeutic relationship. *Journal of Psychology and Counselling*, *1*(2), 30–38.

Barr, W., Hodge, S., Leeven, M., Bowen, L., & Knox, P. (2012). Emotional support and counselling for people with visual impairment: quantitative findings from a mixed methods pilot study. *Counselling and Psychotherapy Research*, *12*(4), 294–302. https://doi.org/10.1080/14733145.2012.663776

Bickenbach, J. E., Chatterji, S., Badley, E. M., & Üstün, T. B. (1999). Models of disablement, universalism and the international classification of impairments, disabilities and handicaps. *Social Science and Medicine*, *48*(9), 1173–1187. https://doi.org/10.1016/S0277-9536(98)00441-9

Billow, R. M. (2000). Self-disclosure and psychoanalytic meaning: a psychoanalytic fable. *Psychoanalytic Review*, *87*(1), 61–79.

Bloomgarden, A., & Mennuti, R. B. (2009). *Psychotherapist revealed: Therapists speak about self-disclosure in psychotherapy*. Routledge.

Bond, T., Griffin, G., Jamieson, A., & O'Dowd, J. (2013). *Ethical framework for good practice in counselling and psychotherapy*. BACP House.

Borg, M. B. (2005). "Superblind": Supervising a blind therapist with a blind analysand in a community mental health setting. *Psychoanalytic Psychology*, *22*(1), 32–48. https://doi.org/10.1037/0736-9735.22.1.32

Bottrill, S., Pistrang, N., Barker, C., & Worrell, M. (2009). The use of therapist self-disclosure: Clinical psychology trainees' experiences. *Psychotherapy Research*, *20*(2), 165–180. https://doi.org/10.1080/10503300903170947

Bridges, N. A. (2001). Therapist's self-disclosure: expanding the comfort zone. *Psychotherapy: Theory, Research, Practice, Training*, *38*(1), 21–30. https://doi.org/10.1037/0033-3204.38.1.21

Britton, R. (1994). The blindness of the seeing eye: inverse symmetry as a defense against reality. *Psychoanalytic Inquiry*, *14*(3), 365–378. https://doi.org/10.1080/07351699409533991

Burke Valeras, A. M. (2007). *To be or not to be disabled: Understanding Identity processes and self-disclosure decisions of persons with a hidden disability* [Ph.D.] Arizona State University.

Calonico, L. D. (1995). *Professional experiences of therapists with physical disabilities* [Ph.D.] California School of Professional Psychology.

Carew, L. (2009). Does theoretical background influence therapists' attitudes to therapist self-disclosure? A qualitative study. *Counselling and Psychotherapy Research*, *9*(4), 266–272. https://doi.org/10.1080/14733140902978724

Charmaz, K. (1995). The body, identity and self: Adapting to impairment. *The Sociological Quarterly*, *36*(4), 657–680. https://doi.org/10.1111/j.1533-8525.1995.tb00459.x

Chernin, P. (1976). Illness in a therapist—Loss of omnipotence. *Archives of General Psychiatry*, *33*(11), 1327–1328. https://doi.org/10.1001/archpsyc.1976.01770110055004

Coren, A. (2010). *Short-term psychotherapy: A psychodynamic approach*. Palgrave Macmillan.

Cozby, P. C. (1973). Self-disclosure: A literature review. *Psychological Bulletin*, *19*(2), 73–91. https://doi.org/10.1037/h0033950

Cubbage, M. E., & Thomas, K. R. (1989). Freud and disability. *Rehabilitation Psychology*, *34*(3), 161–173. https://doi.org/10.1037/h0091722

Farber, B. A. (2006). *Self-disclosure in psychotherapy*. Guilford Press.

Finlay, L. (1999). Applying phenomenology in research: Problems, principles and practice. *The British Journal of Occupational Therapy*, *62*(7), 299–306. https://doi.org/10.1177/030802269906200705

Fitzerman, B. (1996). Anger - The hidden destroyer: A psychodynamic approach with the physically disabled. *Psychodynamic Counselling*, *2*(3), 356–375. https://doi.org/10.1080/14753639608411285

French, S. (1995). Visually impaired physiotherapists: Their struggle for acceptance and survival. *Disability & Society*, *10*(1), 3–20. https://doi.org/10.1080/09687599550023697

Freud, S. (1912). Recommendations to physicians practising psycho-analysis. In J. Strechey (Ed.), *The standard edition of the complete psychological works of Sigmund Freud* (Vol. 12, pp. 111–120). Vintage.

Freud, S. (1940). Splitting of the ego in process of defense. In J. Strechey (Ed.), *The Standard edition of the complete psychological works of Sigmund Freud* (Vol. 23, pp. 271–278). Vintage.

Goffman, E. (1963). *Stigma: Notes on the management of spoiled identity*. Penguin.

Goodley, D. (2011). Social psychoanalytic disability studies. *Disability & Society*, *26*(6), 715–728. https://doi.org/10.1080/09687599.2011.602863

Groneck, J. R. (2013). *Hidden in plain sight: Ordinary and extraordinary experiences of vision loss*. MA Communication, Northern Kentucky University.

Grzesiak, R. C., & Hicok, D. A. (1994). A brief history of psychotherapy and physical disability. *American Journal of Psychotherapy*, *48*(2), 240–250.

Hansen, J. A. (2008). Therapist self-disclosure: Who and when. *Dissertation Abstracts International: Section B, Sciences and Engineering*, *69*(3–B), 1954.

Henretty, J. R., & Levitt, H. M. (2010). The role of therapist self-disclosure in psychotherapy: A qualitative review. *Clinical Psychology Review*, *30*(1), 63–77. https://doi.org/10.1016/j.cpr.2009.09.004

Hernandez, M. (2011). *People with apparent and non-apparent physical disabilities: Well-Being, acceptance, disclosure and stigma* [Ph.D.] Alliant International University.

Hobson, R. F. (1989). *Forms of feeling: The heart of psychotherapy*. Routledge.

Jacobs, M. (1998). Seeing and being seen in the experience of the client and the therapist. *European Journal of Psychotherapy & Counselling, 1*(2), 213–230. https://doi.org/10.1080/13642539808402310

Jacobs, M. (2004). *Psychodynamic counselling in action*. Sage.

Jeffery, M. K., & Tweed, A. E. (2014). *Clinician self-disclosure or clinician self-concealment? Lesbian, gay and bisexual mental health practitioners' experiences of disclosure in therapeutic relationships* [online]. Counselling and Psychotherapy. Retrieved August 21, 2014, from https://doi.org/10.1080/14733145.2013.871307

Joseph, B. (1985). Transference: The total situation. *International Journal of Psychoanalysis, 66*(4), 447–454.

Jourard, S. M. (1971). *The transparent self*. Van Nostrand Reinhold.

Kleege, G. (1999). *Sight Unseen*. Yale University Press.

Kuusisto, S. (1998). *Planet of the blind*. Faber & Faber.

Lane, R. C., & Hull, J. W. (1990). Self-disclosure and classical psychoanalysis. In G. Stricker & M. Fisher (Eds.), *Self-disclosure in the therapeutic relationship* (pp. 31–44). Plenum.

Langs, R. (1998). *Ground rules in psychotherapy and counselling*. Karnac Books.

Lemma, A. (2003). *Introduction to the practice of psychoanalytic psychotherapy*. Wiley.

Mallinckrodt, B., & Helms, J. E. Effect of disabled counselors' self-disclosures on client perceptions of the counselor. (1986). *Journal of Counseling Psychology, 33*(3), 343–348. https://doi.org/10.1037/0022-0167.33.3.343

Maroda, K. J. (2010). *Psychodynamic techniques: Working with emotion in the therapeutic relationship*. Guilford Press.

Merleau-Ponty, M. (1968). *The visible and the invisible: Followed by working notes*. Northwestern University Press.

Miller, M. J. (1991). Counselors with disabilities: A comment on the special feature. *Journal of Counseling and Development, 70*(2), 347–349. https://doi.org/10.1002/j.1556-6676.1991.tb01613.x

Moore, J., & Jenkins, P. (2012). 'Coming out' in therapy? Perceived risks and benefits of self-disclosure of sexual orientation by gay and lesbian therapists to straight clients. *Counselling and Psychotherapy Research, 12*(4), 308–315. https://doi.org/10.1080/14733145.2012.660973

O'Connell, C. T. (2011). *Self-disclosure and the disabled psychotherapist: an exploration of how psychotherapists with visible physical disabilities or differences speak to their clients about these issues*. Massachusetts School of Professional Psychology.

Olkin, R. (2002). Could you hold the door for me? Including disability in diversity. *Cultural Diversity & Ethnic Minority Psychology, 8*(2), 130–137. https://doi.org/10.1037/1099-9809.8.2.130

Parker, C. A. (2011). Religious self-disclosure in informed consent describing a pragmatic and pluralistic psychodynamic approach. *Dissertation Abstracts International: Section B: The Sciences and Engineering, 71*(9–B), 5801.

Peterson, Z. D. (2002). More than a mirror: The ethics of therapist self-disclosure. *Psychotherapy: Theory, Research, Practice, Training, Spring, 39*(1), 21–31. https://doi.org/10.1037/0033-3204.39.1.21

Phillips, A. (2012). *Missing out: In praise of the unlived life*. Hamish Hamilton.
Pizer, A. (2016). Do I have to tell my patients I'm blind? *Psychoanalytic Perspectives*, *13*(2), 214 229. https://doi.org/10.1080/1551806X.2016.1156435
Segal, J. (1993). Against Self-Disclosure. In W. Dryden (Ed.), *Questions and answers on counselling in action* (pp. 10–14). Sage.
Segal, J. (1996). Whose disability? Countertransference in work with people with disabilities. *Psychodynamic Counselling*, *2*(2), 155–166. https://doi.org/10.1080/14753639608411271
Segal, J. (2006). Working psychodynamically with people with physical illness or disability. *Psychodynamic Practice*, *12*(2), 127–129.
Shakespeare, T. (1994). Cultural representation of disabled people: dustbins for disavowal? *Disability & Society*, *9*(3), 283–299. https://doi.org/10.1080/09687599466780341
Shakespeare, T., & Watson, N. (2002). The social model of disability: An outdated ideology? *Research in Social Sciences and Disability*, *2*, 9–28.
Shapiro, J. L. (1990). *Parameters of self-disclosure among psychodynamic and humanistic therapists* [Ph.D.] Long Island University.
Smith, J. A., Flowers, P., & Larkin, M. (2009). *Interpretative phenomenological analysis: Theory, method and research*. Sage.
Spencer, M. (2000). Working with issues of difference in supervision of counselling. *Psychodynamic Counselling*, *6*(4), 505–519. https://doi.org/10.1080/13533330050197115
Stanley, N., Ridley, J., Harris, J., & Manthorpe, J. (2011). Disclosing disability in the context of professional regulation: A qualitative UK study. *Disability & Society*, *26*(1), 19–32. https://doi.org/10.1080/09687599.2011.529663
Stricker, G., & Fisher, M. (1990). *Self-disclosure in the therapeutic relationship*. Plenum.
Thurston, M. (2010). An Inquiry into the emotional impact of sight loss and the counselling experiences and needs of blind and partially sighted people. *Counselling and Psychotherapy Research*, *10*(1), 3–12. https://doi.org/10.1080/14733140903492139
Thurston, M., McLeod, J., & Thurston, A. (2013). Counselling for sight loss: using systematic case study research to build a client informed practice model. *The British Journal of Visual Impairment*, *31*(2), 102–122. https://doi.org/10.1177/0264619613481777
Vick, A. L. (2007). *(Un)settled bodies: A visual phenomenology of four women living with (in)visible disabilities* [Ph.D.] University of Toronto (Canada).
Wachtel, P. L. (2011). *Therapeutic communication: Knowing what to say when*. Guilford Press.
Watermeyer, B. (2012). Is it possible to create a politically engaged, contextual psychology of disability? *Disability & Society*, *27*(2), 161–174. https://doi.org/10.1080/09687599.2011.644928
White, A. (2011). There by the Grace of.... *Therapy Today*, *22*(5), 10–14.
Wilson, S. (2003). *Disability, counselling and psychotherapy: Challenges and opportunities*. Palgrave Macmillan.
Wilson, S. (2006). To be or not to be disabled: The Perception of Disability as Eternal Transition. *Psychodynamic Practice*, *12*(2), 177–191. https://doi.org/10.1080/14753630600655538
Winnicott, D. W. (1971). *Playing and reality*. Tavistock.
Yoshino, K. (2007). *Covering: The hidden assault on our civil rights*. Random House.

How might psychotherapy improve its service to disabled people and people with physical impairment?

Sally Parsloe

ABSTRACT

This article considers how psychotherapy might better serve disabled people and people with physical impairment. Psychotherapy stands accused of making things worse for people living with physical impairment. Exploration of the articulation by Freud and Lacan of the emergence of subjectivity reveals the reason for the distrust of the disability studies community. However, a call has been made for psychotherapy to reflect, reform and be of service. Aspects of psychotherapeutic philosophy stand ready to offer a meaningful response; phenomenology as elucidated by Heidegger, Levinas' notions of alterity and the primacy of the other, and the unravelling of meta-narratives provided by post-modernism and post-structuralism. These aspects, together with the will to self-critique, offer a way of working that moves to an appropriate respect and service from psychotherapy for disabled people.

I want to propose that psychotherapy could be at the forefront of guarding human subjectivity and that it holds a duty to attempt this for everyone. However, the practice and theory of psychotherapy stands accused of failing the significant number of people who are disabled. In this paper I explore the origins and certain aspects of psychoanalytic thinking to explain why this might be so, and to consider other aspects that might help psychotherapy to improve in the service of disabled people and people with physical impairment.

No more than the therapeutic endeavour can be defined can the person with us in the room. The other is always absolutely different. This ungraspable nature of the other in the alterity described by Emmanuel Levinas (Levinas, 1989, pp. 47–53) demands acknowledgement and respect. In light of that, what I am doing in this paper might seem to go against individual experience, but there is something here about acknowledging that lived experience in the world invokes certain self-identifications, which are not in themselves defining or totalizing. I want to write with particular regard to disabled people and those having a physical impairment.

In writing this paper, I remember my grandfather, gassed in the First war and for whom breath was a luxury, my father, wounded in the Second war and in pain most of his adult life, my grandmother whose arthritis meant limited mobility and pain, my mother who lives with myasthenia and osteoporosis, my uncle and father-in-law with Parkinson's Disease. I remember the child at Brownies, whose psoriasis covered her with terrible skin scales, whose hopeful eye and outstretched hand I and other Brownies avoided. I remember my clients with bodily impairment. I don't have to 'remember' my own experience of body-in-the-world as I feel the pain and discomfort of just sitting upright as I write this piece.

People who come to therapy bring their lived experience, themselves against the backdrop of their lives; the families, social and political structures, the place on the planet, the bodies they were born into, their idioms of thought and speech. It is the responsibility of the psychotherapist to hear every aspect of the person in the room in awareness of the complexity of the task, a task so fluid, unexpected and complex that neither the person nor the therapist can define it.

Psychotherapy and the theorization of disability historically have had an uneasy relationship. This, as Watermeyer puts it, is surprising. *'One would imagine that cultural and personal aspects of bodily difference would be important to a discipline concerned with human subjectivity*'. (Watermeyer, 2013, p. 58). Psychotherapy stands accused by disability studies of remaining aloof from disability, of failing to offer an alliance, of failing to take account of a significant aspect of human experience, and worse, of actively exacerbating the situation of those people who have bodily impairment (Gordon, 1995; Figlio & Richards, 2002; Frosh, 2006 among many others). Indeed Davis (Davis, 2016, p. 8) posits Freud as '*producing a eugenics of the mind*'.

However there have been calls from the realm of disability studies to reconsider psychotherapy as having something to offer. '*Constructive engagement is the only option,*' as Watermeyer puts it. (Watermeyer, 2013, p. 2)

It is incumbent on psychotherapy actively to respond to this call. For some, particularly social model disability theorists (a model that describes people as being disabled by societal factors adverse to people with impairment of the body) (Disability Rights UK Factsheet, 2022) the individualistic nature of therapy might be seen as an amputation of the client from their world, leading inevitably to a vacuum of understanding. What emerges from that lens is that we can only help the client if we are prepared to get down into the scrum of everyday existence, the disturbing quiddity of the world, rather than remaining in the ivory tower of psychoanalysis or distributing mechanical behaviour alteration therapies.

We cannot understand what things mean to people unless we listen to what they describe, allowing space for the client to experiment with the articulation of their experience without imposing ourselves. This is the essence of the therapeutic endeavour. More controversial perhaps is what we allow into the room from the world outside. I want to suggest that we bring also a careful listening to the world that the client and we inhabit, a world which has, as Foucauldian analysis (Foucault, 1976, 1979) reveals, messages, laws, commands, addresses, interpretations, interpellations, power constructions, aggressions and fears that do not show themselves, remaining hidden but energetic in the creation and determination of personal experience. These hidden lines of energy that criss-cross the ether and pierce and string us all are manifested in many ways, for example buildings with stairs.

Words are also the carriers of invisible messages. Disabled, impaired, non-normative, restricted, such words are indications not only of characteristics of particular bodies, but designations of societal and political positionings of those characteristics. Are not all human bodies restricted in some manner? Most people can't run like Usain Bolt. Most people can't jump higher than their own knees from standing. Most people can't lift more than 10 kilos with one hand. These restrictions do not invoke the epithets disabled or impaired. The clue is in the 'most people'. It is the deviation from the norm that marks out the suspect body. Lennard J Davis (Davis, 2016, p. 1) says, '*To understand the disabled body one must return to the concept of the norm, the normal body*'. He goes on, '*The "problem" is not the person with the disabilities: the problem is the way that normalcy is constructed to create the "the problem" of the disabled person'.* In thinking about norms however, it must be recalled that there are around 14 million disabled people in the UK (Scope, 2020) and many more have physical impairments that may not invoke a classification of disabled.

It is intrinsic to the bell jar model of mapping (described by Davis as '*the symbol of the tyranny of the norm*' (Davis, 2016, p. 3)) that where there is 'normal', or most occurring, there will be deviations at either end. Sometimes the deviations towards one end are seen as a curse, and at the other blessings; fastest, strongest, tallest, slimmest, most symmetrical, super-abled as opposed to dis-abled. But not too far to the end of the line. Tall is good, too tall is bad. I think of Diane Arbus' photographs of too tall/too short, entitled 'Jewish giant and Mexican dwarf'. These and other of her works provoke stares, an opportunity to ogle a differentiated body without 'causing offence' or bringing yourself into disrepute. These bodies have slipped beyond appearance that evokes merely a passing glance. A further twist is that same physical characteristic in different people is seen differently. A young person who walks with a stick is disabled, but an eighty-year-old with a stick is designated elderly and goes un-noticed. A woman of five foot one is not seen as ridiculous but a man of that same height who dares to assert himself is subjected to the jibe 'small man syndrome'. A bald woman in the street will attract stares, a bald man will not. An infant that waves its little arms involuntarily is cute, an adult doing the same is shocking. And what of the people whose restrictions don't show in the same way as those with visible impairment, people say with chronic illness? Interpretation of the diverse body is a point of view.

Particular embodiments then are seen in such a way that over and above any inherent physical characteristic or function, they have imposed upon them a narrative of the signification of that characteristic, and that imposition operates from and through '*an embedded curriculum of signs, overt communications and assumptions which identify bodily impairment as the central signifier which shapes the social destinies of disabled people*'. (Watermeyer, 2013, p. 29)

Within disability studies different modalities provide different narratives. The medical model is the lens of curing, repairing, bodily non-normativity as sick, the impaired as unhealthy, incomplete, unwholesome. The social model is the view of disability as created by the normative world, a world constructed inevitably which does not fit all people, indeed excludes many. How has bodily impairment been narrated by psychotherapy?

Freud wrote about people who were suffering from physical ailments that had as their origin disturbances of the psyche, but not much about people who had medically diagnosed embodied restrictions that were 'organic'. There were no clients in wheelchairs, no blind clients, no people with MS or cystic fibrosis or Lupus or lacking arms. He was interested in *'the enigmatic condition which, from the time of ancient Greek medicine, has been known as "hysteria" and which has the power of producing illusory pictures of a whole number of serious diseases.'* (Freud, 1909/2013, p. 5)

He explored the implications of impairment through this lens. There is in his output however, a little paper called 'The Exceptions'. (Freud, 1916, pp. 309–333). Here he talks about how the doctor asks his patients *'to make the advance from the pleasure principle to the reality principle by which the mature human being is distinguished from the child'*. Freud observes that there are certain people who deem themselves exceptions to the need to make this advance. Who are these people?

'I succeeded in discovering a common peculiarity in the earlier experiences of these patients' lives. Their neuroses were connected with some experience or suffering to which they had been subjected in their earliest childhood, one in respect of which they knew themselves to be guiltless, and which they could look upon as an unjust disadvantage imposed upon them'.

Freud confirms who exactly he has in mind by citing as an example of these exceptions Shakespeare's Richard III, *'a figure in whose character the claim to be an exception is closely bound up with and is motivated by the circumstance of congenital disadvantage'.*

Having established the connection between disabled people and an inability to move away from childhood to maturity, he goes on to indicate that it is love, as well as the ups and downs of life that enable a person to move from being an 'incomplete human being' to this maturity. One cannot doubt the conclusion of this paper, the exceptions, those who don't submit to his cure, are incomplete humans and destined to immaturity and lovelessness.

Just as one is on the cusp of hurling his paper across the room, Freud comes up with one of his insights. *'And now we feel that we ourselves might become like Richard, that on a small scale, indeed, we are already like him. Richard is an enormous magnification of something we find in ourselves as well'.*

Freud tells us (Freud & Strachey, 1962, p. 26) that the ego is a bodily ego, a representation of the body, and his use of the Richard III character confirms this idea. Freud recognises what it is in us that Richard reminds us of, the corrosive bitterness of reproach for primal past wounds unsurmounted by passage into a maturity that the psychoanalytic cure provides, and which prevents the satisfactory resolution of ego formation so that in Richard and others like him, the ego is arrested in its primary narcissism, in unfinished emergence, touchy, vulnerable and malign.

Unfriendly reference to disabled people is located in another of Freud's papers. In 'The "Uncanny"' (Freud, 1919, pp. 217–256) Freud discussed an undefinable feeling that we sometimes get. *'The subject of the "uncanny" . . . undoubtedly belongs to all that is terrible – to all that arouses dread and creeping horror; it is equally certain, too, that the word is not always used in a clearly definable sense, so that it tends to coincide with whatever excites dread'*. (Freud, 1919, p. 217). The association between the uncanny and bodily impairment is made in part because of Freud's linking of the sensation with images of amputation, '*dismembered limbs, a severed head, a hand cut off at the wrist, feet which dance by themselves, these have something peculiarly uncanny about them*' (Freud, 1919, p. 244). He ruminates on various possible understandings and implications of the uncanny, noticing that the German translation is Unheimlich, with the opposite being Heimlich, and discovering that these two seeming opposites have the capacity to blend into each other in usage, '*Thus heimlich is a word the meaning of which develops towards an ambivalence, until it finally coincides with its opposite, unheimlich*'. (Freud, 1919, p. 223). Heimlich, he discovers, can also mean that which should be kept hidden, a secret, the unspeakable. He expands into the concept of the double, the doppelganger, that which is like oneself, but not oneself, an image from which he draws an association with the idea of the ego and the superego, that which looks from itself at itself. Its quality of uncanniness Freud attributes to the creation of this double dating back to a mental stage long since left behind and forgotten, and the creation of a superego that crushes free will and restricts the ego; the creation of the accusatory like-us-but-not-us, was-us-but-no-longer-us, is the fundamental creation of restriction. Freud suggests '*If this is indeed the secret nature of the uncanny, we can understand why the usage of speech has extended das Heimliche into its opposite das Unheimliche; for this uncanny is in reality nothing new or foreign, but something familiar and old – established in the mind that has been estranged only by the process of repression. This reference to the factor of repression enables us, furthermore, to understand (the) definition of the uncanny as something which ought to have been kept concealed but which has nevertheless come to light*'. (Freud, 1919, p. 236). In other words, a morbid anxiety repressed but which recurs. The most powerful anxieties and infantile complexes, Freud says, are around death- dead bodies, or beings that we can't decide are dead or alive (Olympia in Hoffman's The Sand-Man), the like us but not like us- and the castration-complex, cyphers of which Freud articulates in this paper as dismembered limbs, a severed head, a hand cut off at the wrist, Oedipus' blinding of himself, eyes pulled out of heads, bleeding eyes, madness, epilepsy. He speaks (in relation to the castrated) of '*the horror of the mutilated creature or triumphant contempt*'. (Freud, 1925, p. 252).

I want to suggest that the uncanny is about what is in us or what we used to be that we can't bear to think about, an echo of the unpleasant realisation that '*we ourselves are like Richard*', a reminder of our primal mental state of narcissistic helplessness, of the vulnerability of the body, the ego and of our very subjectivity. Those realities are too much for us. Death is ourselves not ourselves, an incomprehensible, indescribably absolute nothing, solitude, silence. Castration is a terrifying mutilation, a visceral stand in for the ripping away of power, self and meaning, helplessness, death and castration as the ultimate restrictions.

The story of Oedipus Rex could be interpreted in a very different way if one recalls Oedipus having suffered a violent injury as a child (hobbled at the ankles by his father), leaving him with bodily impairment. Oedipus was able to read the riddle of the Sphinx, the answer being ‘a man walking with a cane’. It is the understanding of a man who himself walks with a cane. It his experience of his own bodily limitation, damage, pain and need for assistance that enables him to see, just as it is the blindness of Tiresias that enables him to see what for others with 20/20 vision will always be dark. On the revelation of Oedipus’ shame, he chooses to blind himself, and it is this self-mutilation, this link between bodily impairment, punishment and shame that is chosen to be the focus of the tragedy, not the link between impairment and wider understanding. The self-mutilation of Oedipus is equated with castration, a powerlessness symbolised by the non-phallic human being, the un-symbolisable human. Disabled people, the incomplete, women, and finally all ‘other’ are positioned outside and deviant. Imputation is made that they must be bitter about their exile from the universal and therefore carry malign intent towards the complete- the hegemonic world, a premise made by Freud in The ‘Uncanny’, ‘*Whoever possesses something at once valuable and fragile is afraid of the envy of others, in that he projects on to them the envy he would have felt in their place . . . and when a man attracts the attention of others by noticeable, and particularly by unattractive, attributes, they are ready to believe that his envy is rising to more than usual heights and that this intensity in it will convert it into effective action*’. The crux of the Freudian metanarrative is underpinned by a horror of castration *and the castrated*. The Freudian connection between the castrated and disabled people positions them as objects of fear because of their supposed envy, as well as objects of contempt. No wonder Wilton (2003, p. 372) asks ‘*to what extent is psychoanalysis itself implicated in the reproduction of anxieties surrounding disabled bodies?*’

The analysis of the formation of the ego by Jacques Lacan (Lacan, 2007, pp. 75–81) is also built on an image of the body-in-pieces. Lacan’s description of the moment of the emergence of subjectivity rests on the moment of the infant surging towards its own reflection in the mirror. The infant encounters an image of itself as complete, in contradiction to the fragmented, inchoate, uncontrollable ‘inside’ that it experiences. The baby recognises the image in the mirror as the ‘Ideal-I’. The infant is not able to support itself from its own body, being held up by a parent, or a baby walker. The infant is ‘trapped in motor impotence and nurseling dependence’, by the ‘malaise and motor uncoordination of the neonatal months’. The I is cast in a dichotomy between what it is and what it appears to be. The subject becomes inevitably alienated from itself, and even in therapeutic reflection can only achieve partial realisation, never resolution, of that alienation. The illusion of unity is fixed on the image of the unified body. The unconforming body in Lacan's theorization as well as in Freud's dares to remind us of what we disavow to protect the ego.

The disability theorist Mollow (2018) reiterates that Lacan describes disability in a manner that lends a hand to the notion of the unwelcome signifiers that the impaired body holds and how it can't be tolerated.

> Although Lacan does not refer here to any particular impairment-rather he envisions a non-disabled child passing through a normative developmental process- his language evokes commonplace representations of disabled bodies. One effect of Lacan's essay, then is to suggest that the process of ego formation is inseparable from a fantasy of transcending disability. (Mollow, 2018, p. 171)

Reminders of our own fragmented nature, vulnerability and mortality must be 'put' somewhere. Where do we, as therapists, put people who cause us a frisson of unpleasant jouissance, the equivalence of Freud's uncanny, the very representation of what we fear for and in ourselves? Like it or not, as therapists, we are all the children of Freud, even in our reaction formations. It is from that heritage that the accusation of disability theorists against psychotherapy has justifiably grown, but which may also enable articulation of the charge against itself, as discussed by Wilton (Wilton, 2003).

I have described the way in which the psychoanalytic lens can be unhelpful when thinking about the non-conforming body, but I want to suggest that it carries the potential to be uniquely helpful if it can rigorously self-critique. When this self-critique lapses the world of the client is lost and the possibility of understanding dislocated. The wheelchair user Joshua Smallweed demands in Dickens' Bleak House 'Shake me up, somebody, if you'll be so good'. Do we as therapists need to be shaken up? Progress has been made. For example, aspects of thoughtful working are described in the BACP publication 'Working with disability across the counselling professions' (Halacre, 2020). More is still to be done.

Other ways of shaking it up may be through post-modernism and post-structuralism. Meta-narratives are the core of modernism. One narrative might be the psychoanalytic narrative of the mind described by Freud. Others might be social and medical models of disability.

Post-modernism aims to achieve a shift in knowledge and culture while post-structuralism argues that subjects are embedded in and created by a complex network of social and political relations that determine which subjects may appear, where and in what capacity. If we think through these concepts (elaborated by, among others, the Frankfurt group) we see that no narrative of disability can be the final word, the complete account. There will always be something excluded. Mollow (2018) particularises this facet of narrative in raising the risk that the social model, helpful in challenging the medical model of disability, could deny aspects of bodily impairment that are in themselves problematic, aside from being problematized, like pain or fatigue. If disability is interpreted as existing because the world has failed, as it indubitably has, to accommodate people who can't climb stairs, hear, see, sit upright, speak, hold a cup, type or carry stuff, what then happens with the problem of pain? For many people pain, fatigue, feeling queasy and ill are daily features of life, or features that flare up unpredictably and restrict aspects of living. The social model can address some aspects of this, but not all. For example, my job involves sitting and listening. Since an injury, sitting comes with pain and this isn't going to go away. Sometimes, when it's bad, I lie down to see the clients. Some of them are amused by this inversion, them in the chair and me on the couch. Some don't like it and complain, some are angry, some concerned, but we co-use it as material. I have to be honest and say my bodily pain restricts me in my work in some ways, say the number of people I can see in a day, but it enables a creativity with the people I can see. It restricts me from doing things I used to do easily before. Some time ago, a person with Parkinson's Disease said to me he felt like he had what he termed embodied restriction, and sometimes that's how I feel. I experience an embodied restriction.

Narratives may establish hierarchies of disability that incorporate or exclude certain people. Who is disabled, and who is not? What words may we use to describe our experience of our embodied self in the world? Which narrative is being related, what angle are we coming from, what investments have we got, what are we protecting? These are essential interrogations. Self-interrogation, though essential, is only the beginning. Awareness of theories, narratives, diagnoses and presumptions, including our own, that surround the client is awareness of what gets in the way of hearing the client without our own complexes and those of the world drowning the client out. Garland-Thomson calls for '*A strategic essentialism, which validates experience and consciousness, imagines community, authorises history, and facilitates self naming.*' (Garland-Thomson, 1997, p. 283). This seems to me to be a call to phenomenology.

Phenomenology takes us to the quiddity of the client, which includes their experience of the world into which they are born. From Being and Time, (Heidegger, 1927/1962, p. 60/36) we find that phenomenology means '*to let that which shows itself be seen from itself in the very way in which it shows itself from itself*'. Heidegger is talking about the thrownness into the world of our existence. We are beings in the world. '*Dasein understands its own Being [. . .] in terms of that entity towards which it comports itself proximally*', (BT 36; 15–16). Heidegger's philosophical idea was to let being be (although in practice he supported a totalitarian system that gassed to death bodily unconforming people). By letting being be, by allowing the client to be, to describe and re-describe their life in their own words, the client is able to experience themselves as they are situated in the world. The motto of disability activism comes to mind 'Nothing about us without us'.

Heidegger made a distinction (BT 157–159) between two different ways in which we care for human beings, intervening care and anticipatory care. The first is where we jump in and take decisions for people, and the second is respecting the other's integrity and capacity, getting out of the way of the client to create an opening for their existence with all their limitations and possibilities, to show themselves as they are and to develop in accordance with their own circumstances and freedom. What's it like? is the question phenomenology poses.

Getting out of the way of the client is an initial part of our obligation to the client. For Levinas, our responsibility goes much further. The other person is absolute alterity, never 'like us' or 'like we might become' and *therefore* worthy of care, but an alterity that always comes first, always already comes before us. I venture to suggest that this is not a philosophy widely implemented in the world, as we see the world's many failures respectfully to accommodate diversity. In the therapeutic room, working phenomenologically, we aim to give the client space to describe, but the project of 'understanding' and 'knowing' is, through the other's difference, impossible, unless in a totalizing glance that eradicates them. It is the face of the other that calls to a fundamental ethics of responsibility, not pity, which latter, since Aristotle, has been the foundation of Western moral philosophy. Levinasian 'othering' is an opposite concept to the modern common usage with all its hostility to difference. Although Levinas uses the terms compassion and pity, he distinguishes between these as moral sentiments, that which we 'ought' to have, and compassion as describing the weight of the substitutive responsibility to the primacy of the suffering other (Levinas, 1998, p. 94). Levinas' thoughts are put into pithy reflection in the motif 'Piss on pity' deployed by the disability rights activist Alan Holdsworth in the 90's when protesting against the patronising image of disability in the Telethon TV production. Before the possibility of autonomous choice about 'helping', the primacy of the other, the existing other, calls for a compassion that '*can be affirmed as the very nexus of human subjectivity, to the point of being raised to the level of supreme ethical principle*'. (Levinas, 1998, p. 81)

Disclosure statement

No potential conflict of interest was reported by the author.

References

Davis, L. J. (Ed.). (2016). *The disability studies reader* (5th ed.). Routledge.

Disability Rights Factsheet. (2022). https://www.disabilityrightsuk.org/social-model-disability-language

Figlio, K., & Richards, B. (2002). Psychoanalysis in the public sphere: Some recent British developments in psychoanalytic social psychology. In R. Hinshelwood & M. Chiesa (Eds.), *Organisations, anxieties, and defences: Towards a psychoanalytic social psychology* (pp. 183–203). Whurr Publishers.

Foucault, M. (1976). *Birth of the clinic: An archaeology of medical perception.* Tavistock.

Foucault, M. (1979). *Discipline and punish: The birth of the prison* (A. Sheridan, Trans.). Vintage Books.

Freud, S. (1916). Some character-types met with in psycho-analytic work: The exceptions. The Standard Edition of the Complete Psychological Works of Sigmund Freud, Volume XIV (1914–16): On the History of the Psycho-Analytic Movement, Papers on Metapsychology and Other Works, 309–333.

Freud, S. (1919). The uncanny. The Standard Edition of the Complete Psychological Works of Sigmund Freud, Volume XVII (1917–19): An Infantile Neurosis and Other Works, 217–256.

Freud, S. (1925). Some psychical consequences of the anatomical distinction between the sexes. The Standard Edition of the Complete Psychological Works of Sigmund Freud, XIX: 248–258.

Freud, S. (2013). *Five lectures on psychoanalysis.* Read. (Original work published 1909)

Freud, S., & Strachey, J. (1962). *The ego and the id.* Norton.

Frosh, S. (2006). *For and against psychoanalysis* (2nd ed.). Routledge.

Garland-Thomson, R. (1997). Feminist theory, the body, and the disabled figure. In L. Davis (Ed.), *The disability studies reader* (pp. 279–292). Routledge.

Gordon, P. (1995). Private practice, public life: Is a psychoanalytic politics possible? *Free Associations, 5*, 275–288.

Halacre, M. (2020). *Good practice across the counselling professions 007. Working with disability across the counselling professions.* British Association for Counselling and Psychotherapy.

Heidegger, M. (1962). *Being and time* (J. Macquarrie & E. Robinson, Trans.). Harper and Row. (Original work published 1927)

Lacan, J. (2007). *Ecrits* (B. Fink, Trans.). WW Norton.

Levinas, E. (1989). *The Levinas reader.* Blackwell.

Levinas, E. (1998). Useless Suffering. In M. Smith & B. Harshav (Eds.), *Entre Nous: Thinking-of-the-other* (p. 81). Columbia University Press.

Mollow, A. (2018). Lacan and disability studies. In A. Mukherjee (Ed.), *After Lacan: Literature, theory and psychoanalysis in the twenty-first century* (p. 171). Cambridge University Press.

Scope. (2020). *Disability facts and figures.* Retrieved November 2, 2020, from www.scope.org.uk/media/disability-facts-figures

Watermeyer, B. (2013). *Towards a contextual psychology of disablism.* Routledge.

Wilton, R. D. (2003). Locating physical disability in Freudian and Lacanian psychoanalysis: Problems and prospects. *Social & Cultural Geography, 4*(3), 369–389. https://doi.org/10.1080/14649360309069

Towards an integrative model of multicultural responsiveness

Daryl Mahon

ABSTRACT

There is an increasing need for practitioners to be responsive to multicultural identities in clinical practice. Although the multicultural competency framework has been around for a number of decades, its overall utility and generalisability has not being consistently established. The book chapter approach to learning about multicultural engagement is rather limited, not least because it is impossible to learn about the vast identities of the different cultures that the average practitioner will work with in routine practice. In response to this gap in the literature, the current paper proposes an integrative model of multicultural responsiveness that brings together trans-theoretical practices from the extant literature. In doing so, this paper provides a model of multicultural practice that seeks to learn about the client's complex multicultural identity during the assessment phase, during therapy, and by monitoring the process and outcome of care. A case vignette is provided demonstrating the application and utility of this model.

Introduction

Multicultural responsiveness is an essential part of effective therapy. Drawing on five individual but interconnected concepts three of which are multicultural specific; multicultural orientation, explanatory health model, and intersectionality; and two transtheoretical interventions, preference accommodation, and feedback informed treatment, I describe how practitioners can become responsive to diverse multicultural identities in the therapeutic environment. This integrative model is presented as building on the multicultural competency literature through an integration of independent and interconnected interventions from the extant literature. In the first section of this paper, an overview of the multicultural competency literature is provided.

Then, the five domains of the integrative model are outlined, before moving on to illustrate their application and utility with a case vignette. Firstly, a brief description of the five domains is provided to the reader.

Intersectionality is a theoretical framework for understanding how aspects of a person's social and political identities combine to create different modes of discrimination and privilege. For example, gender, caste, sex, race, class, sexuality, religion, disability, and physical appearance (Crenshaw, 1994). Multicultural Orientation (MCO) is a framework for assisting practitioners to be responsive to cultural identities. The three components are cultural humility, cultural opportunities, and cultural comfort. The Explanatory Health model is an anthropological concept that situates the personal understanding of illness and possible treatment pathways within a cultural context. Preference Accommodation is used to assess clients' preferences as they relate to treatment type, mode, and other important factors to do with treatment. Finally, Feedback Informed Treatment is an approach to improving the quality and effectiveness of treatment through monitoring the process and outcome of care. This integrative model aims to offer a brief multicultural approach that practitioners can use to be responsive to diverse multicultural populations and intersectionality. It can be assimilated into current practices with relative ease and some basic training.

Overview of the multicultural competency literature

The multicultural competency (MCC) movement can be considered the fourth force in psychotherapy, following on from the psychodynamic, behavioural and humanistic traditions (Pedersen, 2002). The competency movement has gained increasing attention since the 1980's across settings such as psychiatry, psychology, therapy and social work.

MCC proposes that it is possible to learn to work with diverse client populations across cultures, identities and treatment paradigms by adapting treatment to specific cultural identities. However, concerns have consistently been noted within the extant literature regarding the extent to which diversity has been included in research trials of evidence-based therapies, and the extent to which these therapies are effective for those from diverse ethnic and racial population (Huey & Polo, 2008; Huey et al., 2014; Miranda et al., 2005; Sue et al., 1992). Disparities in mental healthcare treatment have also been consistently identified within racial and ethnic minority groups, and studies have documented that many practitioners have better outcomes with white clients (Drinane et al., 2016; Hayes et al., 2015; Imel et al., 2011).

While researchers have attempted to respond to these issues, overall the evidence has been mixed as to the effectiveness. Indeed, some research studies have demonstrated that cultural tailoring can sometimes diminish the impact of general practice (Huey et al., 2014). While the MCC approach has seemed to garner most attention, Huey et al. (2014) suggest that there are questions concerning its applicability and effectiveness in general. In addition, there is little support for the position that MCC are a stable characteristic of the practitioner, as studies have not illustrated adequate convergence across ratings of the same practitioner (Owen et al., 2011), or that competencies are strongly linked to outcomes. This is not surprising when we contextualise it within the general outcome research in counselling. That is, the correlation between therapist competency and client outcomes is weak, with less than 1% of the variance in therapy outcomes accounted for by competency (Wampold, 2015; Wampold & Imel, 2015; Webb et al., 2010). Thus, employing another competency framework for cultural counselling may not be the most effective method to improve client outcomes.

Instead, a 'way of being 'discussed later as multicultural orientation (Owen et al., 2016) in sessions is proposed, which would be more aligned to the factors set out in evidence based relationships (Norcross & Lambert, 2011; Norcross & Wampold, 2018, 2019).

The MCC approach stipulates three broad ideas:

- That there are a set of competencies that can impact client outcomes and can be acquired by therapists through a standardised training regime.
- Competency in these skills can be assessed and identified in the therapist.
- The competencies are a standard characteristic across client populations.

Smith et al. (2011) in a meta-analysis of 65 quasi/experimental studies found that culturally adopted treatments had a medium effect size of ($d = 0.46$), with treatments adopting metaphors/symbols that match the clients cultural worldview and treatments to specific ethnocultural identities being more effective. However, for the author this may only be a fruitful approach for those working with ethnocultural demographics, practitioners would have to learn an insurmountable amount of treatment approaches with specificity to work with the variety of intersectional multicultural identities who attend routine practices. At the same time, many of the studies in this meta-analysis did not test direct comparison, thus caveats apply.

That is, interventions were not compared against other bona fide treatments, rather waiting list and non-active controls were used, meaning effect sizes are found to be larger, due to not having bona fide comparisons. Similarly, Griner and Smith's (2006) meta-analysis found that treatment adapted to specific cultural identities was as much as four times as effective (d = 0.45), and matching clients to therapists who speak their own language were up to twice as effective. Again, this may be helpful for working with ethnocultural populations, but practitioners may not find this an approach that can be generalised to routine practice with a more diverse population of clients, or indeed, when intersectionality is more pronounced for a client.

In their meta-analysis, Benish et al. (2011) found that culturally adapted psychotherapy for race/ethnicity is more effective than un-adapted (d = 0.32) compared against bona fide therapies. Adaptation of the illness myth (explanatory health model) was the sole moderator of superior outcomes via culturally adapted psychotherapy. The smaller effect size when analyzed against the above Smith study may be accounted for by the fact that direct comparisons (bona fide treatments) were used. Thus, this effect size is a more accurate picture of effectiveness in a comparative context. Huey et al. (2014, p. 1) in their Annual Review of Clinical Psychology, posit that 'support for cultural competence as a useful supplement to standard treatment remains equivocal at best'. However, they do note the findings from the Benish et al. (2011) study and the adaptation of the explanatory model and it's link to relational common factors. In addition to noting some of the findings from the Smith et al. (2011) meta-analysis, specifically, matching worldview, metaphors and symbols. The explanatory health model adaptation would seem to be congruent with the general psychotherapy outcome variance literature, that suggests building expectancy, hope and providing a rationale for treatment outcome/credibility, produces superior outcomes (Constantino, Coyne, et al., 2018; Constantino, Vîslă, et al., 2018; Frank & Frank, 1991; Wampold, 2015; Wampold & Imel, 2015).

It is for these empirical reasons that the explanatory model is incorporated into this integrative approach (Figure 1).

Tao et al. (2015) meta-analysis of multicultural competency examined MC and its correlation with several processes and clinical outcomes. Specifically, MC was correlated with process measures (r = .075) and clinical outcomes (r = 0.29). The analysis in this study suggest that client ratings of practitioners' MC account for approximately 37% of the variance in the therapeutic alliance, 52% of the variance in client satisfaction, 38% of the variance in general competency, and 34% of the variance in session depth.

Thus, Tao et al. (2015, p. 344) suggest that 'therapist MC should be considered an important empirically supported therapeutic relational factor', with a variance of approximately 8.4% on outcomes. The findings from this meta-analysis provide a good foundation for including Feedback Informed Treatment with its focus on process and outcome measures, in this integrative approach.

Integrative multicultural responsiveness model

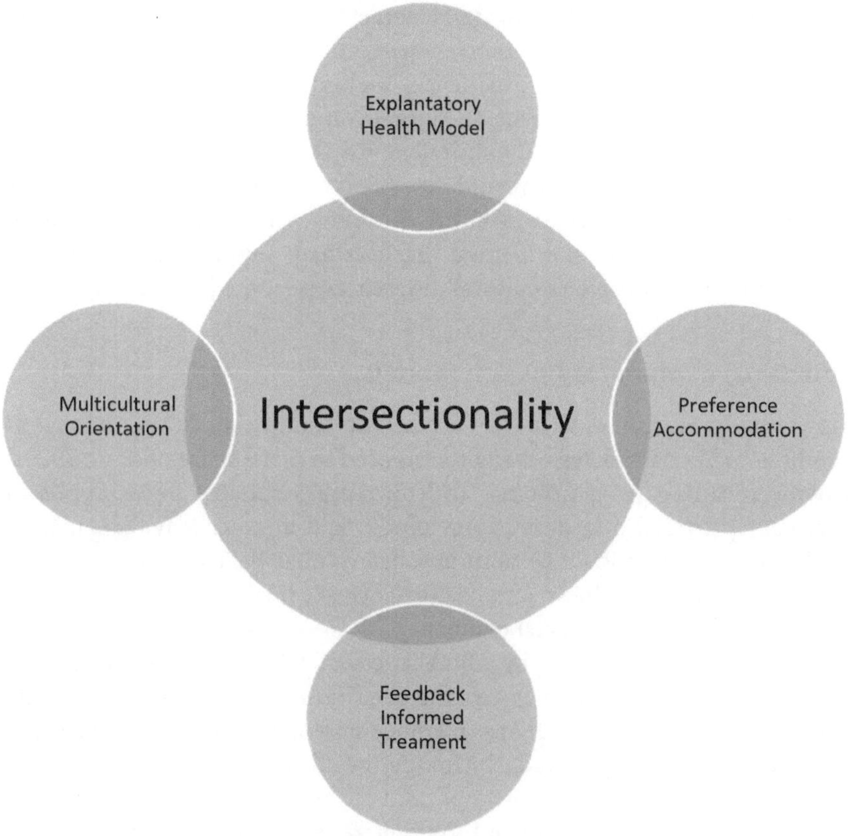

Figure 1. Illustrates each domain of this integrative model.

Domain 1. Intersectionality

Intersectionality is a theoretical framework for understanding how aspects of a person's social and political identities combine to create different modes of discrimination and privilege. For example, gender, caste, sex, race, class, sexuality, religion, disability, and physical appearance (Crenshaw, 1994). Clients are likely to have intersections of and multiple cultural identities, which may all be significant to their lives. As such, it is important for practitioners to not make assumptions about any one aspect of a clients' identity, but rather seek to learn about the contexts in which different aspects intersect and become more prominent in the therapy encounter. For example, within group differences can often be more pronounced than between group differences. Take two individuals sharing the same race, the intersect of sexuality, socioeconomic status or gender can provide for very different experiences of racial identity.

As such, intersectionality provides the practitioner with a theoretical framework and awareness of how different intersecting identities may be more or less impactful to the client's experience. Viewed under this lens, it become quite apparent how the language of cultural competency can be problematic.

As our own privileges and culturally encapsulated existence provide us with huge limitations in understand others, both in terms of practice and the type of research we privilege. Cultural humility, (discussed later in multicultural orientation) is one method that can help support practitioners to become more responsive to cultural differences (George et al., 2020).

Domain 2. Explanatory health models

According to Kleinman et al. (1978) the explanatory models is defined as a complex, culturally determined process used to make sense of one's illness, provide meaning to symptoms, and to express suitable expectations of treatment provided and desired outcomes. Said another way, explanatory models can be described as culturally determined beliefs that individuals hold about suffering, illness, and health. They are mediated by the illness, in addition to cultural and social contexts.

These models are shaped by, and shape societal expectations of the sick role, individual illness and help-seeking behaviour. As such, the acceptability of different treatment paradigms, methods and approaches will vary based on the culturally encapsulated explanatory health models each person views the world through. Hence, it is important for practitioners to acknowledge the explanatory model and attend to it where indicated. The exploration of the explanatory model by the practitioner can help to shape interventions and treatment approaches, while also impacting positively on outcomes for mental health difficulties (Benish et al., 2011; Dinos et al., 2017; Kleinman, 1980; Kleinman et al., 2006). For example, when comparing explanatory models of illness among four cultural groups in the United Kingdom; West African, African Caribbean, Bangladeshi and White, McCabe and Priebe (2004) found perceived cause of illness to be different and significantly related to treatment satisfaction.

This would seem to be congruent with the ideas put forward by Benish et al. (2011, p. 281) who postulate that; 'what is important to the sufferer, is not the scientific validity or falsifiability of the illness explanation but rather the congruence of the explanation with the client's cultural beliefs about the illness'.

However, it must be noted that explanatory models are dynamic and can change through various socio-cultural means, including further education and access to new information.

One method of successful culturally informed psychotherapy has been documented by Benish et al. (2011), whose meta-analysis researched the explanatory health model, using the term illness myth to describe it. As far back as 1962, Wrenn described psychotherapy as culturally encapsulated, calling for more cultural diversity in the delivery of treatment. Frank and Frank (1991) and Wampold (2007) suggest that an important aspect of universal healing is the cultural explanation and a set of healing rituals provided to the client which are embedded within a cultural context. Frank and Frank (1991) identified this phenomena many years ago, conceptualising it in the following way;

- A confiding relationship with a culturally recognized and sanctioned healer,
- A context and/or setting distinguished from the ordinary
- A rationale or myth providing a plausible explanation for the illness
- A ritual or intervention believed by both to be an effective means of restoring health

For practitioners, the following key areas based on Rüdell et al. (2008) research can inform the adaptation of the explanatory model as part of the assessment process, and when indicated through the course of therapy. Practitioners can skilfully solicit information regarding some, or all, of the following:

- Inferences about the types of symptoms experienced (somatic, mental, or behavioural).
- Assumptions of the aetiology of the Illness (psychosocial, supernatural, behavioural, natural, physical).
- Estimation of the timeline or course of illness (acute, chronic, episodic).
- Client postulation about consequences resulting from the illness (self, social relationships, economic standing, physical, behavioural).
- Subsequent expectations about what types of treatment would be appropriate.

The adaptation of the explanatory model would seem to be especially important in providing a rationale that is consistent with the clients cultural understanding, beliefs about symptoms, aetiology, how the issues will evolve, and opinions on acceptable treatment approaches. This is not to say that a practitioner must incorporate the client's explanatory model wholesale, but at the very least, a practitioner must be willing to listen before offering their own explanatory explanation, or collaboratively building a new one. Considering the impact that incorporating this has on outcomes (Benish et al., 2011), we find that it is a good fit with a good evidence base for this integrative model.

The explanatory model can be used throughout therapy; however, we see an initial benefit in its use during the assessment phase and it can be used in conjunction with preference accommodation (discussed in domain 3), especially when multicultural needs have been initially identified through administering the Cooper-Norcross Inventory of Preferences. As such, it is a starting point where the practitioner can learn from the client their important cultural identities, how they view their presenting issues, and what, if any, ideas they have regarding treatment within a cultural context.

Domain 3. Preference accommodation

Preference accommodation is based on the idea of pluralism. That is, different people need different things, at different points in time, and that no one approach holds all the answers nor be effective for all people (Cooper & McLeod, 2007). The Cooper and Norcross Inventory of Preferences (2016) is an 18-item brief, multidimensional measure to help clients articulate the style and approach that they desire in counselling. Preference accommodation is a domain in this integrative model as it can capture both latent and manifest cultural beliefs linked to the explanatory health model that can be further unpacked during therapy. There are also questions relating to client preference towards their therapist, across demographics of diversity. While not a cultural specific inventory, it does provide a good starting point to begin incorporating important client preferences in general, which can be explored under a cultural lens also.

This idea, and flexibility, converges nicely with the explanatory model, which itself can be considered as 'cultural pluralism'. That is, clients may have different culturally specific ideas of how treatment should work, and what type of approaches and methods will be helpful. Swift et al. (2018) demonstrate in their meta-analysis that preference accommodation is associated with superior client outcomes and reduced early attrition, both of which have been shown to disproportionately impact clients of diversity.

The cultural implications of research, treatment and our understanding of therapy also need to be carefully considered, least they are not congruent with the client's experience of their emotional problems. While this is important for all people, it comes into sharper focus when we consider diversity. For example, the Western world's diagnostic system of pathologizing, is certainly not consistent with all cultures, nor is the individualistic approach to therapy. Many cultures have a collectivist way of viewing well-being and Western ideas of personal growth and self-actualisation may not be consisting with such worldviews. Our research and training has taught us to re-cast other people's experiences in terms of our own culturally situated symbolic system and this may be problematic for working with some types of diversity. Thus, it will be helpful for the practitioner to have multicultural practices that can be used in the moment, a process orientation as opposed to a competency. Owen et al. (2016) discuss the multicultural orientation as a way to achieve this.

Multicultural orientation

For Watkins et al. (2019) the Multicultural Orientation (MCO) can be viewed 'as a process-oriented, attitudes-additive perspective to the MCC Knowledge Skills and Attitude (KSA) framework'. MCO is used to operationalise the process-oriented perspective and as a complement to the attitudes component of the KSA framework; and the multicultural competency approach in general (Davis et al., 2018). The MCO approach is made up of three interconnected, and interdependent ideas; cultural humility, cultural opportunity and cultural comfort. The orientation approach is more aligned to a process and attitude on the part of the practitioner, therefore, it is not a competency that can be taught through a protocol with fidelity. How a practitioner uses the multicultural orientation will be influenced by many factors such as the values and worldview they hold, experiential avoidance, and their awareness of other cultural dynamics. Davis et al. (2018, p. 90) describes what this process entails 'The cultural worldviews, values, and beliefs of the client and the therapist interact and influence one another to cocreate a relational experience that is in the spirit of healing'.

As such, one practitioners response may look entirely different than another. The following three components of MCO will provide the practitioner with a framework to help guide their practice.

- Cultural humility: Means being aware of cultural and power dynamics that are at play between therapist and the client and approaching these issues without defensiveness but with collaboration (Hook et al., 2016).
- Cultural opportunities are 'markers that occur in therapy in which the client's cultural beliefs, values or other aspects of the client's cultural identity could be explored' (Owen et al., 2016). They occur when clients mention their beliefs, values or other details that provide an opportunity for the therapist to explore the client's cultural identities in more depth.
- Cultural comfort is characterised by feeling at ease, open, calm, or relaxed with diverse others (Davis et al., 2018). As such, cultural comfort refers to the therapist's thoughts and feelings that emerge before, during and after interactions with the client about cultural identities and values.

Cultural humility, can be considered a virtuous component of the MCO approach. Increasingly, those across disciplines within the mental health domains have come to understand humility as an alternative and/or complementary language to the competency approach (Davis et al., 2018; Foronda et al., 2016). Humility is conceptualised as consisting of both intrapersonal and interpersonal components. That is, a level of self-awareness regarding the view a practitioner holds of themselves, and their limitations; and the extent to which one is other orientated rather than being more concerned with having the correct knowledge and answers for the client. We can therefore extrapolate that cultural humility as a subdomain of humility is the extent to which a practitioner can hold an interpersonal position with a client that is curious about their client's cultural identity, and not assuming one knows what meaning is ascribed to such cultural identities. Or as Hook et al. (2013, p. 354) articulate 'the ability to maintain an interpersonal stance that is other-oriented (or open to the other) in relation to aspects of cultural identity that are most important to the client'

Culturally humble therapists seek out markers for cultural opportunities to enquire into clients identities that arise in session. These culturally humble therapists seek to find cultural comfort in these interactions while engaging differential client cultural identities.

While cultural humility seems to be the foundation to this orientation, Watkins et al. (2019) suggests that on its own, it may not be enough to improve outcomes. Importantly, cultural humility goes beyond the traditional position of 'not knowing' adapted by practitioners, and actively seeks to learn from clients, their cultural identities. If cultural humility is the motivational factor for practitioners who want to find out about others important identities, then cultural opportunity and cultural comfort can be considered the in session behaviours when these markers are identified, and need to be broached. Said another way, through cultural humility, practitioners identify important cultural markers as they present in session, and broach the subject using cultural opportunities.

Owen et al. (2016) describe cultural opportunities as those points in a session where important cultural beliefs, values and identities present and can be explored by both practitioner and client. At the same time, cultural opportunities are not always present, and therapists should feel that they can broach these issues if they feel that there will be therapeutic value in situations where cultural opportunities may not be manifest. Davis et al. (2018) suggest doing this gently and authentically and without big transitions or forcing the issue. Hence, practitioners who practice cultural humility and opportunity will have a certain level of ease with engaging in these practices, that is, cultural comfort. Cultural comfort explains the level of ease that practitioners experiences before, during and after conversations with clients about their cultural identities (Owen et al., 2014). While cultural comfort would be needed to navigate the complex interpersonal dynamics that occur in session, cultural discomfort may be a good indication that something has been triggered and needs attending to. As such, Davis et al. (2018) use the language of cultural transference and counter-transference. Viewed under this lens, feelings of cultural discomfort may precede cultural humility and would seem important for practitioners to identify as they may impede therapeutic progress.

The current evidence for MCO in therapy is emerging as strong across a number of studies (Davis et al., 2018; Owen et al., 2014, 2016). Microaggression is a term used to describe commonplace verbal or behavioural indignities, whether intentional or unintentional, that can communicate hostile, derogatory or negative attitudes towards stigmatised or culturally marginalised groups (Sue & Sue, 2016). Owen et al. (2016) found that clients who experienced microaggressions from their therapists experience worse therapeutic alliances and worse therapy outcomes. At the same time, Owen et. al. (2016) found that therapists ability to identify 1 of 3 microaggressions in simulated sessions was 38% to 52%. Hook et al. (2016) demonstrated that for clients who experienced microaggressions, cultural humility predicted the number and impact of these aggression after controlling for general multicultural competencies, indicating the added value of humility.

In a retrospective study, Owen et al. (2016) examined therapist cultural humility and missed opportunities. Findings suggest that clients who rated their therapist as culturally humble had better therapy outcomes, while those who rated their therapist as having missed opportunities to discuss their cultural identity (cultural opportunity) reported worse outcomes. Again, Owen et al. (2014) in a study focused on religious cultural identities reported that therapist who were more culturally humble with religious clients had better outcomes. It's not surprizing that multicultural orientations seem to be mediated by the therapeutic alliance. Hook et al. (2013, study 1) found that cultural humility was correlated with the alliance.

In a second study, Hook et al. (2013, study 2) demonstrated that cultural humility correlated with the alliance and client outcomes. In a third study, Hook et al. (2013, study 3) found that cultural humility mediates the alliance and client outcomes.

Taken together, these seven empirical studies demonstrated positive client outcomes, and thus, the MCO is incorporated into the present integrative model.

Domain 5. Feedback informed care

Feedback Informed Treatment (FIT) is an evidence based trans-theoretical approach for improving the outcome and process of behavioral healthcare

(Miller et al., 2016). FIT involves using two ultra-brief measures at every session to solicit feedback from clients on the therapeutic alliance and outcome of care, and using the information provided to adapt the therapists approach in real time to meet these needs. FIT uses the Outcome Rating Scale (ORS) to solicit feedback on how the client is responding to treatment, that is, the benefit they are getting from therapy. The Session Rating Scale (SRS) is used to assess the therapeutic alliance. Both measures are reliable and valid tools, and their use can improve therapy outcomes by helping to identify those not benefiting from care; at risk of early termination, and those actively deteriorating while in care; all of which make up a significant percent of clients in routine practice. Importantly, the SRS as I discuss shortly, can be utilized for attending to multicultural alliance ruptures.

One of the most cited rationales for clinicians incorporating multicultural competencies into therapy, is how poorly clinicians attend to ethnic and other minorities (Huey et al., 2014), and the disparities within mental health outcomes for these populations. However, individual clinician experiences and opinion may not be congruent with the literature. For example, several studies during the last 30 years (Allison et al., 1996; Hansen et al., 2006; Holcomb-Mccoy & Myers, 1999; López & Hernandez, 1986; Maxie et al., 2006) of predominantly white therapists illustrates that between 72–91% of clinicians perceive themselves as practicing multicultural competencies to some extent. For the author, it is difficult to reconcile these statistics.

While Benish et al. (2011) suggests that this may be reflective of a certain level of cultural competency as a norm, another way to view these statistics could be through the lens of cognitive bias on the part of practitioners. The less knowledge, expertise, and self-awareness one has about a field of practice, the more likely one is to overestimate their degree of knowledge or competency in that area (Kruger & Dunning, 1999). So, having less expertise working with an area of diversity might make it harder for one to see one's limitations in that area. This bias, combined with self-enhancement dispositions, may make it difficult for practitioners to perceive and take responsibility for their limitations (Davis et al., 2018). Indeed, Fuertes et al. (2006), and Dillon et al. (2016) found that counsellor's self-assessment of their multicultural competencies was found to exceed that of their client's assessment. This may not be overly surprising considering the previously cited Owen (2013) study on therapists ability to spot microaggressions as they happen in session.

At the same time, the general psychotherapy literature informs us those clinicians tend to overestimate their rates of client improvement and underestimate their rates of client deterioration (Chow et al., 2015; Walfish et al., 2012). Thus, in the studies cited above, clinicians may be overestimating their abilities and or use of cultural competencies. One method to help practitioners improve these issues is by tracking their progress, outcome, and process of care with standardized measures. Coupled with the previous research attesting to the power of the alliance in multicultural therapy, feedback approaches would seem to be indicated as helpful tools.

Specifically, the SRS can be used to keep track of the therapeutic alliance in general, but also within a culturally informed manner.

As the measure tracks the extent to which clients are satisfied with the bond between themselves and the practitioners; the goals and topics discussed; and the methods and approach used. In doing so, practitioners may also garner a clearer picture of their multicultural abilities and align their process orientation more towards the individual diversity and intersectionality's that their clients present with, reducing possible self-effectiveness bias.

Hook and colleagues (2016) inform us that as many as 81% of clients have experienced at least one microaggression from their therapist. Clients 'who perceive racial – ethnic microaggressions from therapists have reported lower therapeutic alliances and diminished therapy outcomes' (Owen et al., 2016). At the same time, therapists may be unaware of microaggressions that occur in session, thus, tracking the alliance with a structured measure at the end of each session may be one way to identify and attend to cultural ruptures in real time. For example, one type of microaggression, 'colour blindness' can happen when, let's say, a white therapist informs their black client that they don't see them as different. While this can be an attempt by the practitioner to convey to the client that they are a human being of equal worth and importance, it is very often experienced as dismissive of the clients identity. The impact of this is what I refer to as a 'multicultural alliance rupture'.

Considering that all of the empirical studies discussed previously indicated that multicultural outcomes were mediated through the alliance, it makes sense that we explicitly attend to this when working with diversity. Indeed, in their meta-analysis, Tao et al. (2015) suggest that clients' perceptions of their therapists multicultural competency accounts for 37% of the variability in therapeutic alliance. While FIT has a specific meaning regarding feedback, all the domains discussed previously seek feedback from clients in some manner, it is this attitude and willingness to learn from the client, that is at the heart of this integrative model.

Case study

In the following case study, I present this integrative model in a linear format illustrating how it can be used during initial assessment, throughout the therapy process, and in monitoring the process of therapy by paying attention to the therapeutic alliance in a multicultural manner. Importantly, and at the heart of this model, is the idea that each of the four practice components are used to learn from the client's important cultural values, beliefs, and identities, explanatory health model, and how these can inform therapeutic responsiveness from practitioners. While the four practice components are discussed in a linear manner for ease of understanding their application, there is a great deal of overlap in their use during therapy. While the fifth concept, intersectionality, describes the clients' varied cultural identities, which can help the practitioner build awareness of differences that they might not otherwise be aware of due to their own privileges.

Juda is a 36-year-old Sub-Saharan African gay man who has recently arrived in England escaping persecuting due to his sexuality. During the first appointment which was an assessment, Juda was administered the Cooper-Norcross Inventory of Preference. The therapist conducting the initial assessment explained the purpose of the questionnaire to Juda prior to filling it out. While there was no strong preference for a counselling style, the therapist noticed that Juda preferred a female therapist of English origin, in addition to medication to help manage how he is feeling. Coincidentally, the therapist conducting the assessment, Donna, was a White female of English nationality. The therapist was aware of the research demonstrating that matching clients to therapists of similar demographics and cultural identities has shown to be more effective and wanted to inform Juda about this.

Donna: Thanks for completing this questionnaire, Juda, I notice that you prefer a White English female therapist, is this correct?

Juda: Yes, please. I am happy to see you if that is, ok?

Donna: Of course, I would be happy to take you on as a client. However, I know many clients often feel more comfortable with therapists who may have more things in common, such as gender, nationality, or for example, race or sexuality. I'd just like to check to see if this is something that interests you?

Juda: No, please, no. This is not helpful to me!

Comment: At this point in the session Donna was aware of the intersectionality that was present and wondered how this was evolving. Donna was also unsure why the opportunity to have a therapist of similar cultural identity was refused, especially considering the research on its effectiveness. Donna viewed this as a 'marker' that could be used as a cultural opportunity to enquire into Juda's experiences. At the same time, Donna is demonstrating cultural humility by taking a 'not knowing' stance, especially in the face of the research that she is aware of.

Donna: It seems that I have brought up something that will be of little use to you? I was trying to be more helpful, but I suspect that I am off the mark. I'm curious as to the possible reasons for this, can you help me understand?

Juda: In my country, it is criminal to be homosexual. I cannot be who I want to be. I am being punished for my badness, through bad mental health. Even here, in your country, I am seen as a black immigrant and not good enough.

Donna: It's not safe for you to express your identity. This is so unfair, I don't see you as different, you are human, just like me.

Comment: In her effort to convey unconditionality and acceptance, Donna unintentionally 'committed' a microaggression. Donna also became aware that Juda's explanatory model may be an area to explore. The reader will recall the previous points that a practitioner can use to assess the client's explanatory model.

Donna: Juda, I wonder if you can help me understand your experience a bit more? I'd like to hear why you think you are feeling this way, and how this relates to being punished?

Juda: Yes, in my region, homosexuality is a sin, it is the work of sorcery being visited on me. It has corrupted my brain; my mind does not work properly now. This is way I need medication. In my country, I would go to a faith healer, but this is not an option for me. Without medication, my brain will not be fixed, and I will not be able to have relationships with my family. They refuse to see me whilst I am this way. I am happy to be homosexual, but I need to feel ok before I can think about this . . .

Comment: Donna's skillful question based on knowledge of the explanatory health model allowed her to assess Juda's beliefs about the onset, symptoms, consequences, and treatment options. As we can see the explanatory model is dynamic and fluid. However, Donna also found herself a little uncomfortable especially regarding the onset and treatment options of medication discussed by Juda. Cultural discomfort happens quite often, and it is important for practitioners to be compassionate when this occurs, and to lean into the client at these pivotal moments, when the natural feeling may be to withdraw. Donna also felt that there was an opportunity to explore her own explanatory model with the Juda, while also accommodation some of Juda's explanations.

Donna: Your situation is very difficult for you, and you just want some relief and to reignite contact with your family. In our country I cannot prescribe you medication, however, I can make a referral to a medical practitioner who can do this for you, if that is ok?

Juda: Yes, please, this would be great

Donna: Juda, in our culture we view people as being free to express their sexuality however they choose to, our society largely allows for this. I wonder if having to suppress this while being stigmatized by those around you many have contributed to you feeling bad in some way? In this country we do use medication sometimes, but we also find talking therapy to be helpful. If you would like to try this while waiting to see the doctor, I would be happy to continue to see you and offer support . . .

Comment: Donna offered up her own explanatory model in a non-threatening and non-judgmental manner, with an option for Juda to engage with this he wanted to. Towards the end of the session Donna introduced the idea of using feedback using the Session Rating Scale (SRS).

Donna: Juda, research tells us that I can be most helpful to you if our work is aligned, and we have a broad agreement on the type of work we are doing. That is, do we agree on the goals and tasks, approach, and methods, and is the relationship the right fit. Can I ask you to complete this short four item measure which addresses these areas? Please place a mark on each item, where scores to the left represent dissatisfaction and scores to the right represent satisfaction. Just to say, I am not looking for perfect scores, I'm not perfect. But I am really interested in hearing from you, even things that you may not consider hugely significant, but which improving on may make your experience of our work better.

Comment: Juda filled out the SRS and Donna quickly added up the scores. The SRS is scored out of a total of 40 points. There is a clinical cut-off of 36, which is an indicator of those at risk for poor outcomes and early attrition. Juda scored the SRS at 34, indicating that there may be a rupture to the therapeutic alliance.

Donna: Thank you so much for this feedback, Juda, it will help me improve the service that I provide to you. I notice that the relationship item is scored at 5, can you help me understand what this represents?

Juda: Yes, well, earlier on I was trying to explain my experience of being gay, as well as being a black immigrant in a different country. I am not just like you, my experience is very far from your experience, I feel a little invalidated as a gay black man by how you responded to me.

Donna: Ok, thank you so much for bringing this to my attention Juda. Do you have a sense of what a better response from me would look like?

Comment: Using the SRS Donna was able to address the 'multicultural alliance rupture' by attending to Juda's experience and reestablishing the alliance. In addition, this provided Donna with an opportunity to use cultural humility and opportunity.

Discussion and conclusion

Learning about others culture can be quite difficult, not least because what we learn may not be representative of the wider population, re-stereotyping may occur, and outliers are always present. While adapting to specific ethnocultural populations is one way of providing multicultural support, it is beyond the scope of any practitioner to learn about all cultures, and their intersectionality's. It is just not feasible to learn about others important beliefs, values and cultural identities from a book chapter. Therefore, an approach that can be utilised with differential cultures and their intersectionality would certainly be more feasible for the average practitioner. Huey et al. (2014) in their *Annual Review of clinical Psychology* note that approaches to multicultural therapy that have high training needs, complex protocols and substantial costs, that further narrow their applicability to specific demographics are unlikely to be adapted and maintained by clinicians.

Since MCC presented on the horizon over 50 years ago, the idea of multicultural practice has been embraced at different levels by different disciplines and practitioners. Yet, the research literature is often ambivalent on its conceptualisation and effectiveness as it relates to diversity and the outcomes associated with care. At the same time, the multicultural competency has scant evidence to support its consistent effectiveness. Inconsistencies have been demonstrated in the literature, with different studies having different outcomes and practitioners not being consistent with its use as rated by clients. The present paper contributes to the extant literature in several ways. Firstly, it responds to Huey et al. (2014) call for a multicultural approach that is not overly complicated with excessive training regimes, competency based protocols, and financial burdens.

Secondly, it adds to the current body of knowledge in the multicultural arena by moving beyond the MCC approach, adding a 'phased' integrative model that can be used to identify and learn about clients multicultural identities. At the same time, this model distils concepts already within the literature that have meta-analysis support for their individual effectiveness in multicultural domains and related practices.

Thirdly, one of the strengths is that it offers a mechanism to track and monitor the process and outcomes of care. In light of this integrative model having a process orientation, these tracking systems may be especially important for outcomes and the author hypotheses that it could be these aspects that give this model predictive validity over some of its individual components. Finally, the use of measures of the alliance and outcome of care can assist practitioners in maintaining focus with multicultural issues that are important to clients; to repair ruptures in the alliance that may be caused by microaggressions, lack of cultural humility, or missed cultural opportunities.

However, as the SRS fails to ask explicit questions regarding culture and this may be a limitation. Thus, a cultural item could be added to the SRS, or an existing scale should there be one, could be incorporated.

Given that this integrative model it is based on the most recent research trials, we can be confident that some aspects of the model will likely provide for effective multicultural therapy. However, limitations of the present paper are concerned with the lack of primary data to understand if this model is effective in clinical practice. Thus, future research may wish to study it within a clinical environment with primary quantitative data in a randomised control trial (RCT). In order to establish relative efficacy a RCT with established active controls would need to be considered. The MCO model or the explanatory health model would both individually be considered active controls and could provide data regarding the extent to which this integrative model may add value beyond these individual components.

Disclosure statement

No potential conflict of interest was reported by the author.

ORCID

Daryl Mahon http://orcid.org/0000-0002-2519-2155

References

Allison, K. W., Echemendia, R. J., Crawford, I., & Robinson, W. L. (1996). Predicting cultural competence: Implications for practice and training. *Professional Psychology, Research and Practice*, *27*(4), 386–393. https://doi.org/10.1037/0735-7028.27.4.386

Benish, S. G., Quintana, S., & Wampold, B. E. (2011). Culturally adapted psychotherapy and the legitimacy of myth: A direct-comparison meta-analysis. *Journal of Counselling Psychology*, *58*(3), 279–289. https://doi.org/10.1037/a0023626

Chow, D. L., Miller, S. D., Seidel, J. A., Kane, R. T., Thornton, J. A., & Andrews, W. P. (2015). The role of deliberate practice in the development of highly effective psychotherapists. *Psychotherapy*, *52*(3), 337–345. https://doi.org/10.1037/pst0000015

Constantino, M. J., Coyne, A. E., Boswell, J. F., Iles, B. R., & Vîslă, A. (2018). A meta-analysis of the association between patients' early perception of treatment credibility and their posttreatment outcomes. *Psychotherapy (Chicago, Ill)*, *55*(4), 486–495. https://doi.org/10.1037/pst0000168

Constantino, M. J., Vîslă, A., Coyne, A. E., & Boswell, J. F. (2018). A meta-analysis of the association between patients' early treatment outcome expectation and their posttreatment outcomes. *Psychotherapy*, *55*(4), 473–485. https://doi.org/10.1037/pst0000169

Cooper, M., & McLeod, J. (2007). A pluralistic framework for counselling and psychotherapy: Implications for research. *Counselling and Psychotherapy Research*, *7*. doi:10.1080/14733140701566282.

Cooper, M., & Norcross, J. C. (2016). A brief, multidimensional measure of clients' therapy preferences: The Cooper-Norcross Inventory of Preferences (C-NIP). *International Journal of Clinical and Health Psychology*, *16*(1), 87–98. https://doi.org/10.1016/j.ijchp.2015.08.003

Crenshaw, K. W. (1994). Mapping the Margins: Intersectionality, Identity Politics, and Violence Against Women of Color. In M. A. Fineman & R. Mykitiuk (Eds.), *The Public Nature of Private Violence* (pp. 93–118). New York: Routledge.

Davis, D. E., DeBlaere, C., Owen, J., Hook, J. N., Rivera, D. P., Choe, E., & Placeres, V. (2018). The multicultural orientation framework: A narrative review. *Psychotherapy*, *55*(1), 89–100. https://doi.org/10.1037/pst0000160

Dillon, F. R., Odera, L., Fons-Scheyd, A., Sheu, H. -B., Ebersole, R. C., & Spanierman, L. B. (2016). A dyadic study of multicultural counselling competence. *Journal of Counselling Psychology*, *63*(1), 57–66. https://doi.org/10.1037/cou0000118

Dinos, S., Ascoli, M., Owiti, J., & Bhui, K. (2017). Assessing explanatory models and health beliefs: An essential but overlooked competency for clinicians. *BJPsych Advances*, *23*(2), 106–114. https://doi.org/10.1192/apt.bp.114.013680

Drinane, J. M., Owen, J., & Kopta, M. (2016). Multicultural competencies: What are we measuring? *Psychotherapy Research*, *26*(3), 342–351. doi:10.1080/10503307.2014.983581.

Foronda, C., Baptiste, D. L., Reinholdt, M. M., & Ousman, K. (2016). Cultural humility: A concept analysis. *Journal of Transcultural Nursing*, *27*(3), 210–217. https://doi.org/10.1177/1043659615592677

Frank, J. D., & Frank, J. B. (1991). *Persuasion and healing: A comparison study of psychotherapy*. John Hopkins University Press.

Fuertes, J. N., Stracuzzi, T. I., Bennett, J., Scheinholtz, J., Mislowack, A., Hersh, M., & Cheng, D. (2006). Therapist multicultural competency: A study of therapy dyads. *Psychotherapy*, *43*(4), 480–490. https://doi.org/10.1037/0033-3204.43.4.480

George, J. R., Michaels, T. I., Sevelius, J., & Williams, M. T. (2020). The psychedelic renaissance and the limitations of a White-dominant medical framework: A call for indigenous and ethnic minority inclusion. *Journal of Psychedelic Studies*, *4*(1), 4–15. https://doi.org/10.1556/2054.2019.015

Griner, D., & Smith, T. B. (2006). Culturally adapted mental health intervention: A meta-analytic review. *Psychotherapy: Theory, Research, Practice, Training*, *43*(4), 531–548. https://doi.org/10.1037/0033-3204.43.4.531

Hansen, N. D., Randazzo, K. V., Schwartz, A., Marshall, M., Kalis, D., Frazier, R., Burke, C., Kershner-Rice, K., & Norvig, G. (2006). Do we practice what we preach? An exploratory survey of multicultural psychotherapy competencies. *Professional*

Psychology, Research and Practice, *37*(1), 66–74. https://doi.org/10.1037/0735-7028.37.1.66

Hayes, J. A., Owen, J., & Bieschke, K. J. (2015). Therapist differences in symptom change with racial/ethnic minority clients. *Psychotherapy*, *52*(3), 308–314. https://doi.org/10.1037/a0037957

Holcomb-Mccoy, C. C., & Myers, J. E. (1999). Multicultural competence and counsellor training: A national survey. *Journal of Counselling & Development*, *77*(3), 294–302. https://doi.org/10.1002/j.1556-6676.1999.tb02452.x

Huey, S. J. Jr., & Polo, A. J. (2008). Evidence-based psychosocial treatments for ethnic minority youth. *Journal of Clinical Child and Adolescent Psychology: The Official Journal for the Society of Clinical Child and Adolescent Psychology, American Psychological Association, Division 53*, *37*(1), 262–301. https://doi.org/10.1080/15374410701820174

Huey, S. J. Jr., Tilley, J. L., Jones, E. O., & Smith, C. A. (2014). The contribution of cultural competence to evidence-based care for ethnically diverse populations. *Annual Review of Clinical Psychology*, *10*, 305–338. https://doi.org/10.1146/annurev-clinpsy-032813-153729

Imel, Z. E., Baldwin, S., Atkins, D. C., Owen, J., Baardseth, T., & Wampold, B. E. (2011). Racial/Ethnic disparities in therapist effectiveness: A conceptualization and initial study of cultural competence. *Journal of Counselling Psychology*, *58*(3), 290–298. https://doi.org/10.1037/a0023284

Kleinman, A. (1980). *Patients and healers in the context of culture: An exploration of the borderland between anthropology, medicine, and psychiatry*. University of California Press.

Kleinman, A., Eisenberg, L., & Good, B. (1978). Culture, illness, and care: Clinical lessons from anthropologic and cross-cultural research. *Annals of Internal Medicine*, *88*(2), 251–258. https://doi.org/10.7326/0003-4819-88-2-251

Kleinman, A., Eisenberg, L., & Good, B. (2006). Culture, illness, and care: Clinical lessons from anthropologic and cross-cultural research. *Focus*, *4*, 140–141. https://doi.org/10.1176/foc.4.1.140

Kruger, J., & Dunning, D. (1999). Unskilled and unaware of it: How difficulties in recognizing one's own incompetence lead to inflated self-assessments. *Journal of Personality and Social Psychology*, *77*(6), 1121–1134. https://doi.org/10.1037/0022-3514.77.6.1121

López, S., & Hernandez, P. (1986). How culture is considered in evaluations of psychopathology. *Journal of Nervous and Mental Disease*, *174*(10), 598–606. PMID: 3760850.

Maxie, A. C., Arnold, D. H., & Stephenson, M. (2006). Do therapists address ethnic and racial differences in cross-cultural psychotherapy? *Psychotherapy: Theory, Research, Practice, Training*, *43*(1), 85–98. https://doi.org/10.1037/0033-3204.43.1.85

McCabe, R., & Priebe, S. (2004). Explanatory models of illness in schizophrenia: Comparison of four ethnic groups. *British Journal of Psychiatry*, *185*(1), 25–30. https://doi.org/10.1192/bjp.185.1.25

Miller, S. D., Bargmann, S., Chow, D., Seidel, J., & Maeschalck, C. (2016). Feedback-informed treatment (FIT): Improving the outcome of psychotherapy one person at a time. In W. O'Donohue & A. Maragakis (Eds.), *Quality improvement in behavioral health* (pp. 247–262). Springer International Publishing. https://doi.org/10.1007/978-3-319-26209-3_16

Miranda, J., Bernal, G., Lau, A., Kohn, L., Hwang, W. C., & LaFromboise, T. (2005). State of the science on psychosocial interventions for ethnic minorities. *Annual Review of Clinical Psychology, 1*, 113–142. https://doi.org/10.1146/annurev.clinpsy.1.102803.143822

Norcross, J. C., & Lambert, M. J. (2011). Evidence-based therapy relationships. In J. C. Norcross (Ed.), *Psychotherapy relationships that work: Evidence-based responsiveness* (pp. 3–21). Oxford University Press. https://doi.org/10.1093/acprof:oso/9780199737208.003.0001

Norcross, J. C., & Wampold, B. E. (2018). A new therapy for each patient: Evidence-based relationships and responsiveness. *Journal of Clinical Psychology, 74*(11), 1889–1906. https://doi.org/10.1002/jclp.22678

Norcross, J. C., & Wampold, B. E. (2019). Relationships and responsiveness in the psychological treatment of trauma: The tragedy of the APA clinical practice guideline. *Psychotherapy, 56*(3), 391–399. https://doi.org/10.1037/pst0000228

Owen, J. (2013). Early career perspectives on psychotherapy research and practice: Psychotherapist effects, multicultural orientation, and couple interventions. *Psychotherapy, 50*(4), 496–502. https://doi.org/10.1037/a0034617

Owen, J., Jordan, T., Turner, D., Davis, D., Hook, J., & Leach, M. (2014). Therapists' multicultural orientation: Client perceptions of cultural humility, spiritual/religious commitment, and therapy outcomes. *Journal of Psychology and Theology, 42*(1), 91–99. https://doi.org/10.1177/009164711404200110

Owen, J., Tao, K. W., Drinane, J. M., Hook, J. N., Davis, D. E., & Kune, N. F. (2016). Client perceptions of therapists' multicultural orientation: Cultural (missed) opportunities and cultural humility. *Professional Psychology: Research and Practice, 47*(1), 30–37. https://doi.org/10.1037/pro0000046

Owen, J., Tao, K., Leach, M. M., & Rodolfa, E. (2011). Clients' perceptions of their psychotherapists' multicultural orientation. *Psychotherapy, 48*(3), 274–282. https://doi.org/10.1037/a0022065

Pedersen, P. B. (2002). The making of a culturally competent counsellor. *Online Readings in Psychology and Culture, 10*(3). https://doi.org/10.9707/2307-0919.1093

Rüdell, K., & Diefenbach, M. A. (2008). Current issues and new directions in psychology and health: Culture and health psychology. Why health psychologists should care about culture. *Psychology & Health, 23*(4), 387–390. doi:10.1080/08870440701864983.

Smith, T. B., Rodríguez, M. D., & Bernal, G. (2011). Culture. *Journal of Clinical Psychology, 67*(2), 166–175. https://doi.org/10.1002/jclp.20757

Sue, D. W., Arredondo, P., & McDavis, R. J. (1992). Multicultural counselling competencies and standards: A call to the profession. *Journal of Counselling & Development, 70*(4), 477–486. https://doi.org/10.1002/j.1556-6676.1992.tb01642.x

Sue, D. W., & Sue, D. (2016). *Counselling the culturally diverse theory and practice* (7th ed.). John Wiley & Sons.

Swift, J. K., Callahan, J. L., Cooper, M., & Parkin, S. R. (2018). The impact of accommodating client preference in psychotherapy: A meta-analysis. *Journal of Clinical Psychology, 74*(11), 1924–1937. https://doi.org/10.1002/jclp.22680

Tao, K. W., Owen, J., Pace, B. T., & Imel, Z. E. (2015). A meta-analysis of multicultural competencies and psychotherapy process and outcome. *Journal of Counselling Psychology, 62*(3), 337–350. https://doi.org/10.1037/cou0000086

Walfish, S., McAlister, B., O'Donnell, P., & Lambert, M. J. (2012). An investigation of self-assessment bias in mental health providers. *Psychological Reports, 110*(2), 639–644. https://doi.org/10.2466/02.07.17.PR0.110.2.639-644

Wampold, B. E. (2007). Psychotherapy: The humanistic (and effective) treatment. *American Psychologist, 62*(8), 857–873. https://doi.org/10.1037/0003-066X.62.8.857

Wampold, B. E. (2015). How important are the common factors in psychotherapy? An update. *World Psychiatry, 14*(3), 270–277. https://doi.org/10.1002/wps.20238

Wampold, B. E., & Imel, Z. E. (2015). *Counselling and psychotherapy. The great psychotherapy debate: The evidence for what makes psychotherapy work* (2nd ed.). Routledge/Taylor & Francis Group.

Watkins, C. E., Jr., Hook, J. N., Owen, J., DeBlaere, C., Davis, D. E., & Van Tongeren, D. R. (2019). Multicultural orientation in psychotherapy supervision: Cultural humility, cultural comfort, and cultural opportunities. *American Journal of Psychotherapy, 72*(2), 38–46. https://doi.org/10.1176/appi.psychotherapy.20180040

Webb, C. A., DeRubeis, R. J., & Barber, J. P. (2010). Therapist adherence/competence and treatment outcome: A meta-analytic review. *Journal of Consulting and Clinical Psychology, 78*(2), 200–211. https://doi.org/10.1037/a0018912

OPEN ACCESS

Deconstructing humanitarian compassion: Ψ as method

Artemis Christinaki

ABSTRACT

This paper discusses humanitarian compassion within the Derridean notion of hospitality. Reflecting on the age of Imperial Humanitarianism where Evangelists formed administrative missions to save the souls of the slaves in the colonial provinces of Europe, it aims to address the link of compassion with Christianity and colonialism. Setting the Christian scene of humanitarianism, hospitality as a Derridean concept is introduced to depict that compassion and aid work in-between certain 'guest and host' territories. The impossibility of hospitality under these circumstances highlight the play of power relations in which the other is produced. While Derrida argues that hospitality cannot be power-balanced unless the language of the host is deconstructed, psychology in the humanitarian sector performs an 'emotional hospitality' which seeks to extract a story of confession. Ψ as method works to open a discussion on suffering, Christianity, and colonialism as a modern form of conversion: the confession of truth in a psychological discourse. Challenging compassion and aid as constituted in psychological discourse, this paper invites therapists to rethink the contextualisation under which these ideals emerged while introducing a discussion on what the language of psychology 'does' to refugees.

Introduction

As Fassin (2007, p. 508) vividly marks in his paper *Humanitarianism as a Politics of Life* there is 'no war without its humanitarian corridors and its humanitarian workers. And no western military intervention into another country is now without its justification on humanitarian grounds'.

A quick recap on what happened in the northern part of Syria, and how troops from different states (i.e. the United States of America, Turkey, Russia) managed to justify their operation there, may shed some light in the way a military intervention is justified 'on humanitarian grounds' or with a humanitarian façade. Witnessing natural disasters and civilian casualties in war, the final decades of the 20th century came also to witness the rise 'of humanitarian crises' as a feature in the discourse of the international media, interstate entities and non-governmental organisations. From the most recent refugee crisis in Syria, to the Rohingya crisis in Myanmar, the crisis in Afghanistan after the war in 2001, the humanitarian crisis in South Sudan or the crisis in Somalia, interventions are additionally justified on a 'crisis discursive-ground' (Goodman et al., 2017; see also Khiabany, 2016). Seeking to supply aid to victims[1], an institutional apparatus of aid emerged over the second half of the 20th century, composing an aid industry which attempted to designate an essential component of human existence, dignity. 'Dignity [played] a central role in documents and claims related to human rights and ethics and [served] as a primary supplement to physical well-being in humanitarian discourse' (Redfield & Bornstein, 2010, p. 20).

If one starts from the hypothesis that the notion of *crisis* was born in capitalist discourse (and formation) with the increasing social inequalities at global level due to financialisation of global capital, the continuous imperial interventions – as in Middle East and Africa – and rapid environmental degradation (Khiabany, 2016), then it may be argued that one needs to examine what underlies humanitarian crises, humanitarian interventions as well as their compassion to dignity. Since the 1990s a core component of these interventions includes psychosocial aspects of disaster and hence the alleviation of human suffering. Violence, horror, and natural catastrophes having been considered critical incidents for the psyche they have now triggered several humanitarian interventions which include the programme of psychosocial support in their operations.

This paper

Barnett (2011, p. 9) in his book *Empire of Humanity: A History of Humanitarianism*, situates humanitarianism in three ages; Imperial Humanitarianism, Neo-Humanitarianism, and Liberal Humanitarianism. As he observes the ages of humanitarianism are distinguished globally within forces of destruction (violence), production (economy) and protection (compassion). For the first age, Imperial Humanitarianism, colonialism was its force of destruction, commerce its force of production and civilising missions its force of compassion.

Having as a primary signifier Barnett's humanitarian topology, this paper attempts to show that suffering and psychosocial support have a long-lasting relationship that dates as far back as the first age of humanitarianism, Imperial Humanitarianism. Situating humanitarian compassion (Redfield & Bornstein, 2010) in the Derridean notion of hospitality (Derrida, 2000, 2003), it is argued that colonialism, Christianity, and the evangelical movements of salvation, paved the way for a modern form of confession in the 'emotional hospitality' of the psychological discourse; or, what I am calling here: Ψ as method (see Kapsali & Mentinis, 2020; Burman, 2019; Chen, 2010; Mezzadra & Neilson, 2013; Siddiqui, 2017)[2]. The latter is a strategy of reading and envisaging what the role of psychology is in the field of humanitarian and migration studies. Psychology as method in this paper starts as an epistemological viewpoint that allows a critical analysis of humanitarianism's compassion past and becomes a research analytic to offer a perspective on what psychology 'does' within humanitarian compassion in the present. It is an anti-humanist project in the sense of a conceptual and methodological intervention which seeks to rethink compassion outside of humanitarian psychic imperialisms and (non)governmental responses.

Programmes of psychosocial support in humanitarian operations usually comprise of one-to -psychological session, group activities either psychologically informed or recreational with a psychological intonation (psychoeducation) and non-formal educational activities (i.e. learning to speak the local language). In these sessions, psychologists aim to help refugees speak for their experiences, agree on some daily life-targets that would awake them to adjust in the new reality and most importantly listen to a story, which may be a passage to their movement from the humanitarian landscape to a more governmental status. Taking into consideration that refugees do not articulate their suffering in a psychological discourse, as it is a very westernised project of comfort, they are trained to speak in the Other's discourse[3]. Learning to speak a new language, the language of psychology within the neutral zone of humanitarian compassion, an 'emotional hospitality' opens to the psyche, to situate the self efficiently in the new terrain. Scholars from different fields and schools of thought have indicated so far, *the politics of the psychosocial* in-between migration studies. For example, Mohanty (1984) and her paper on *Under western eyes: Feminist scholarship and colonial discourses*, De Vos (2011) on '*The psychologisation of humanitarian aid: skimming the battlefield and the disaster zone*', Mills (2013) on *Decolonizing global mental health. The psychiatrisation of the majority world*, Bistoen (2016) on *Trauma, ethics and the political beyond PTSD* and Kapsali and Mentinis (2018) on *Psychologies of Compliance: Notes on the Psychopolitical Control of Migration.*

Inspired by these authors and drawing from my own experience, as a psychologist, former humanitarian aid worker and a researcher in this field, I aim to critically discuss what the language of psychology 'does' to refugees. Without minimising the importance of legal citizenship and other formal rights for those who have been dispossessed of 'land and freedom', I ally with the Derridean notion of hospitality to highlight that the concept of 'emotional hospitality', as it is performed in humanitarian psychological discourse, opens the way in a modern way of confession – conversion. Challenging compassion and aid as they are constituted in psychological discourse, this paper invites therapists to rethink first the contextualisation under which these ideals emerged in the psychological discourse and second to continue the discussion on the politics of psychosocial support.

Setting the Christian scene: Humanitarian compassion, colonialism and the concept of Derridean hospitality

Humanitarianism grew up from the 18th century onwards, emerging and appearing in European experience. Although the response to the Lisbon earthquake in 1755 and the formation of the Red Cross in 1863 comprise two of its critical junctures, there are two important historical shifts that should be considered. The first is the movement to abolish slavery and the second the efforts of administrators and missionaries to care for colonial populations (Redfield & Bornstein, 2010).

Barnett (2011), as mentioned above, has illustrated the history of humanitarianism in three ages. Suffering, confession and protection go back as far as the first age of humanitarianism, the era of colonialism and imperialism (Imperial Humanitarianism). In contrast to the third age (Liberal Humanitarianism) which belongs to the liberal peace, globalisation and human rights, the 'second wave' of humanitarianism (Neo-Humanitarianism) came to indicate that colonialism and the end of its era would bring progress and modernity alongside a non/inter/and governmental vacuum. Even though humanitarianism at the moment belongs in terms of a linear time modality in the meta-era of the liberal humanitarianism, which means one step beyond the institutionalisation of progress and modernity (civil society is such an example), it encapsulated within its modification some particular idioms of its birth like suffering, protection and confession.

Evangelicalism was the most important development of the first age of humanitarianism and was closely associated with the masses' 'awakening' in the colonial provinces of Europe. The process of awakening was performed in the revival of the emotional life-changing event in which the sinner confessed and begged for salvation. Evangelists had a primary role in it as they believed that the purpose of their life was to serve God, an act which required not only their personal salvation but also the devotion of their life to saving the souls of the others. Evangelicals along with secular elites established organisations and charities aiming to redress every form of oppression. In the back streets of London, they were trying to raise awareness regarding the suffering of the slaves in the colonial outskirts. They were encouraging as many people as possible to identify with the suffering of the Other, demonstrating compassion for all the Lord's living creatures (Barnett, 2011, p. 53–55).

Moving back and forth from the colonial outskirts of northern India and West Africa, the founding abolitionists, being most of them evangelicals, were preaching that all Lord's children should be treated with compassion and respect. Interestingly, though, the notion of respect meant the acknowledgement that slaves were also humans, but not as much humans as the white Christians. The Lord's children were not all fully equal in the name of their Father. They were considered as inferior to the highly civilised missionaries. Fighting for their liberation, re-humanisation and civilisation, abolitionists formed administrative missions to educate the slaves and thus civilise them. At a dinner in 1816, William Wilberforce (as cited in Barnett, 2011, p. 60), a British politician, philanthropist and leader in the abolishing slavery movement 'declared that free slaves would come to appreciate their protected position: "Taught by Christianity, they will sustain with patience the suffering of their actual lot . . . [and] will soon be regarded as a grateful peasantry"'. Non-believers could be saved, and evangelicals had found the mission to atone themselves from the sin of slavery and colonialism. Since slavery was a sin against Christianity, Christianity could civilise the slaves initiating them in the doctrine of confession and religion.

In the age of Imperial Humanitarianism, compassion emerged in the name of salvation and civilisation. Confessing their sins, slaves were entering the House of God, admitting their will for salvation. Their confession was witnessing not only their will to be saved but also to be civilised. As humanitarian modification was taking place within the main forces of capitalism's acceleration, the global economy and the ideologies regarding the state's role in society, humanitarian compassion reflected accordingly the economic and the social ferment. Wars as an economic and social rupture in capitalism's formulation and capital accumulation gave prominence to the role of humanitarianism and its compassion.

Oliver (2017) in her paper *Earthquakes: Deconstructing Humanitarianism*, highlights that international humanitarian aid and humanitarian war operate not only as two sides of the same coin but also as two sides of the same sovereign. While wars may be a threat to the sovereign, they sustain both the sovereign and the business of humanitarian aid. As Oliver (2017, p. 39) sarcastically emphasises 'war creates refugees and then we wage more war to address the situation'. Isn't that the case of Syria for example? People fled seeking refuge in neighbouring countries (Turkey, Lebanon, Jordan, Egypt) and Europe mobilised humanitarian assistance while an ongoing military invasion-operation continued taking place in the name of humanitarian assistance. The case of Afghanistan is also a profound example of what an operation may mean in-between humanitarian assistance.

> [T]here is no hospitable house. There is no house without doors and windows. But as soon as there are a door and windows, it means that someone has the key to them and consequently controls the conditions of hospitality. There must be a threshold. But if there is a threshold, there is no longer hospitality. (Derrida, 2003, p. 14)

Hospitality in the dressed-up formation of a 'safe space', along with other provisions of basic human rights such as food, water and access to health care, comprises one of the cornerstones of humanitarian discourse. Without underestimating the significance of these rights and believing in principle that people should have access to them, the aim here is to shift our gaze to the dialectics of this hospitable agency. Oliver, for instance, drawing on Derrida's notion on 'non-hospitable house' makes a crucial link between humanist discourses of tolerance, forgiveness, and hospitality and their Christian roots of sovereignty. In Ephesians II, St. Paul says 'you are no longer foreigners abroad, you are fellow-citizens of the Saints, you belong to the House of God' (as cited in Oliver, 2017, p. 42). The concept of hospitality is inherited from the Christian tradition, depicting a male sovereign mastery of one's own house, family, country and unavoidably country and nation (Oliver, 2017). Compassion and aid work in between these 'guest and host' territories signifying a constitution of hospitality within a play of power relationships.

The way, therefore, we welcome refugees to adjust in a western psychological discourse in which they need to perform their trauma(s), vulnerabilities, and – most significantly – their life-stories based on which they will claim a refugee status, gives rise to a 'self-limitation' as well as a 'self-contradiction' in the form that humanitarian and state hospitality take place (Oliver, 2017). The impossibility of hospitality according to Derrida, the fact that 'there is no hospitable house' signals the constitution of roles between a guest and a host. If humanitarian aid is the host in-between a state agency, then refugees should be considered as guests. However, it is worth noting here that the word hospitality as it unfolds in these roles carries itself a contradictory essence. Hospitality . . .

> . . . derives from the Latin *hospes*, which is formed from *hostis*, which originally meant a 'stranger' and came to the meaning of the enemy or 'hostile' stranger (*hostilis*) + pets (*potis, potes, potential*), to have power. (Derrida & Caputo, 1997; as cited in Nayak, 2015, p. 105)

Hence, the constitution of refugees as guests in a certain territory signifies not only the limitations of hospitality itself but it also encapsulates within it forms of power in the way humanitarian compassion is performed. Linking both with their Christian traditions may signal a House of God in which a refugee may indeed find shelter, but to enter and be accommodated, will need to confess.

Confession and psychology: Building an Emotional House of God

Humanitarianism, as well as Christianity and colonialism, was shaped in different forms and modes as capitalism was emerging. Humanitarianism, for instance, in its most recent form has been performed as an institutional formulation of peace and conflict. Such changes accompanied how the appeal of Christianity slowed down while colonialism was constantly transforming into different modes of racism, secularism, institutional whitening and pseudo-scientific objectivism(s).

Whatever 'progress' has been made since then, there is a core-element that remained almost the same, the *education as a mechanism of conversion*. The latter is what, in my opinion, links humanitarianism-suffering and the modern form of confession inspired by a pedagogical and psychological apparatus.

While missionaries believed that people in Africa could be made to fit into civilisation by changing their spirituality and moral codes (see Vaughn, 1991), psychosocial support in the humanitarian discourse promised an awakening from the life-threatening events that occurred in refugees. Now confessing their stories, like they were their sins, refugees ask for salvation. They ask for opening a case in their asylum service to save their soul by claiming refugee status and let the hospitality begin. While Evangelists were central to slaves' salvation, believing that the purpose of life was to serve God by saving the souls of themselves and others, the modern Evangelists have been re-born via a psychological apparatus that pushes refugees to confess almost saliently and silently their stories to book a room in another House of God. Nevertheless, it is not only their confession that matters, but also the way they learn to speak about themselves as they enter in an Other's House and discourse. It is this form of pedagogy in the psychological discourse that makes education work as a mechanism of conversion and psychology as a method. Every time they confess, the language of psychology teaches them how to speak better and more consistent about themselves as if the language of psychology is the practice of education in a more civilised discourse.

Foucault (1976/1978, p. 53–73) in the first volume of *History and Sexuality* discussed *scientia sexualis* as a civilised practice in the West. Speaking about sex, he argued, interfered between two modes of production of truth: confession and scientific discursivity.

In the Western societies of the Middle Ages, confession was established as one of the main rituals in the production of truth. The evolution of the word *avowal* was emblematic in the development of the legal discourse because it signified that someone was aware of his own actions and thoughts. Admitting your awareness while you confess your truths inscribed as one of the most important techniques in the production of truth and signalled the heart of power in an individualised procedure. In this way, while Foucault unfolds how sex was a privileged theme of confession from the Christian times to his present day, the transformation of revealing a refugee's story into discourse are perhaps two elements of the same deployment.

It is in the act of confession that truth in suffering and compassion are joined through the detailed expression of an individual secret of life. Confession, as a ritual, enforces the speaking subject to make a statement and become *the subject of statement*. Deploying a confession, refugees become the subject of statement in the presence of an inter-governmental partner who is the interlocutor between suffering, humanitarian compassion and state approval. Truth serves as a medium between suffering and compassion and unfolds an interplay of power dynamics. The inter-governmental partner as the host in-between a humanitarian and state territory invite the guest to confess so the hospitality may begin. While truth is guaranteed in the speaking subject and in the evidence that brings along in the discourse of his statement, the agency of domination does not lie in the one who confess but in the partner who listens. Having set the scene under which the hospitality will take place, the discourse of truth takes effect. As Foucault (1976/1978, p. 62) argued, though, its effect does not lie in the one who receives the statement of truth but 'in the one from whom is wrested'.

From the outskirts of North India and West Africa, the evangelical reformation of the eighteenth century came to accompany the nineteenth century medical transformation. The latter encompassed the anticipation of building a science of the subject where experience could work as evidence and introspection as validity. Although there is nothing inherently sinful for both experience and introspection, the medical transformation attempted to constitute them as a way of functioning of truth in society. The science of the subject emerged in the medical transformation as an individualised power who came to establish not only a new way in the inscription of truth but also the relational way in which it will be inscribed. In other words, it established a different version of the 'host-guest' relational schema in the performativity of 'humanitarian compassion -in- refugee' or 'psychology -in- patient'.

The combination of confession with examination of suffering in the humanitarian psychological appraisal (see the case of PTSD: Bistoen, 2016; Summerfield, 1997, 1999), the personal history with the deployment of certain signs and symptoms, the formulation of specific tools for identifying psychological distress (see for instance Marquer et al., 2012) and the recollection of memories in the refugees' representation in the humanitarian discourse all constitute ways of re-inscribing the procedure of confession in the field of humanitarian and scientifically approved psychological discourse. Deploying your story became a theoretical tool of confession which had to be thorough, meticulous and coherent. Its consistency mattered not only to operate in the scientific discourse of the psychologist or the lawyer who participate in the procedure of claiming status, but also in the recognition that humanitarian discourse performs compassion.

Nevertheless, compassion cannot be expressed if one solely confesses. Hosting compassion means to console and direct the work of documenting the truth in order to pass through the validation of claiming a status. As Foucault (1976/1978, p. 67) states, 'the obtaining of the confession and its effects were recodified as therapeutic operations'. Thus, the life story of the refugee is no longer accounted for a simple inscription of truth in the claiming of the status, but it started inscribing the boundary between the normal and the pathological, or to put it in another way the expression of compassion in a psychologised discourse. The psychotherapeutic turn of humanitarian aid, taking place in the 1990s as a response to the crisis of humanitarianism (Pupavac, 2004) implied that suffering from now on would derive its meaning and its necessity from the psycho-medical discourse in the programmes of psychosocial support. As Pupavac (2004, p. 497) demonstrates, this psychosocial turn may have attempted to 'bring back the human in the face of the bureaucratisation of aid, foregrounding how people and communities personally experience disaster or conflict', but it also situated psychological discourse as an important mode of effective nature in trauma's alleviation as well as effective adjustment of the self in the new conditions of living.

The *scientia sexualis*, Foucault argued, emerged in the 19th century and reserved its primary element of recognition as 'the singular ritual of obligatory and exhaustive confession'. The latter was a technique that the Christian tradition employed to produce the truth of sex. It may be argued then, that the pedagogy in the psychological discourse is what makes *education* work as a mechanism of conversion and psychology as a method. Teaching refugees how to speak about themselves through the deployment of a story, the introspection of their traumas and the introvert expression of their experiences are both a method and a form of *conversion* in the psyche of the western territory (see also Parker, 2007). Confession is what converts them into guests in the western host's territory as well as its discourse. Every time they confess, they learn how to speak better the discourse of the Other, the psychological discourse, which also gives them access in the national territories of the Other. Psychologising their experiences, educating them to speak a new language and creating an alternate House of God in-between therapeutic discourses reflect on what the notion of psychosocial comprise in the humanitarian terrain. It does not therefore come as a surprise that most of the humanitarian personnel in the current operation in Greece consist of psychologists, social workers and educators.

Migrating from the backstreets of Imperial Humanitarianism, Neo-Humanitarianism, Liberal Humanitarianism and its new forms embracing progress and modernity shifted, if not transformed, the forms of salvation. Nowadays, the safe space of a refugee camp is not considered the Lord's

House. Rather it is established as a mobile clinic in a so-called neutral host's territory which offers a moment of peace that will come through confession. Psychologists, as Evangelists and abolitionists, could not save the modern slaves of capital if they do not express the wish to free themselves (Barnett, 2011). Instead, to free someone and recognise him as a guest, there has to be a story to be told, a story that will certify that indeed you have experienced a number of sins which you confess and you can now move into the Emotional House of God: humanitarian compassion, psychology and salvation. It is along these lines that 'emotional' hospitality takes place and psychology as method performs.

Humanitarian compassion as an emotional hospitality: Ψ as method

Derrida proposed rethinking immigration within the field of conditional hospitality. The latter is offered primarily by governments and occurs in the name of property. Penelope Deutscher (2003, p. 9) argues that a gesture of hospitality asserts someone's right to approve or forbid access as well as occupation in a nation's land. In this way the host is also the gatekeeper who has the power to decide who may pass or not. In the case of the current 'refugee crisis', offering hospitality to refugees was one of the many means by which European governments displayed their ownership over the territory which refugees were crossing, and in which have been offered residency or restriction of access. However, it was not only the state that performed as the gatekeeper of this territory but also the actors of humanitarian aid. United Nations High Commissioner for Refugees (UNHCR), the International Organisation for Migration (IOM), or the Red Cross have worked closely with European governments to provide aid amid the 'refugee crisis'. Sharing the burden and the role both of the gatekeeper and the host, they had the authority to document refugees as soon as they arrive in the country, guide them in the process of seeking refuge and applying for asylum and accommodate them in certain national territories which have been offered by the state. In this process, Ψ professionals have a key role while they work hand in hand with the host's law. National and European legal procedures inform and direct psychosocial interventions and have an impact on the terms and conditions of hospitality (i.e. Greek legal asylum procedures, Dublin II). Although, it is not the purpose of this paper to explore the relation of psychology with these legal procedures, it is important to note that law creates certain conditions for the hospitality of refugees, and psychology performs as one of its methods.

Taking into consideration that many humanitarian operations consist of local agents (Fassin, 2007, p. 515–516), which belong and indeed may represent the interest of the national host, the notion of Derridean hospitality does not only take place in terms of territorial access and citizenship laws but also in the psychic capability of the 'guest' to embody a presence in another's land of dwelling. Questions around identity, life story, reasons of migration and ability of adaptation perform in everyday humanitarian discourse to provide a *raison de être* in this national landscape. It is in this performative action of confession, of admitting why 'you are here and not there', that suffering, confession and psychology interplay, signalling a new form of sovereign power and a modern form of conversion: the confession of truth in a humanitarian psychological discourse.

Derrida (as cited in Deutscher, p. 9, see also Derrida, 1999) has indicated that 'the position assumed by the "hospitable person", the adjudication, the granting of passage, the assertion of authority to grant or deny access is itself inherently inhospitable'. A true hospitality according to him, would require 'the invention not only of its own forms, rules, or conditions *but also of its own language*'. Elaborating on the notion of the Derridean hospitality and its performative character in the figures of 'the host and the guest', I claim that humanitarian compassion as it is encompassed in the performance of psychosocial support creates a space of 'emotional hospitality' which is inherently *in*hospitable.

Humanitarian organisations mediate in the process of othering refugees in a monolingual perspective. Programmes such as *psychosocial support* train refugees to confess their story and learn how to speak about themselves in the language of the Other. Emotional hospitality is the space where the language of psychology unfolds as the language of the Other. Psychology as method mediates in the way refugees learn to deploy their experiences and initiates them in the process of introspection. The articulation of their experience in the language of the Other and their ability to perform introspection constitute the counter pillars of making their life-story functioning as truth in the process of seeking refuge. Every time the story will be confessed, a form of awakening takes place. The awakening of the self in the psychological discourse lies in the work of *psychology as method* because it proves the credibility of the self in the deployment of the story.

As refugees learn how to speak about what happened, they are initiated in a psychological discourse which not only will give them access to claim status but may also be the threshold to move from one territory to another. In the case of Greece, for example, the way your vulnerabilities will be deployed, it may be the passage of movement from the islands to the mainland or from the refugee camps of the mainland to an urban accommodation project. Psychological language is *a form of monolingualism* in the sense that the way you learn to speak about your symptom 'proves' your own awakening/Enlightenment/worthiness to the Other. You confess in the language of the Other.

Inspired by Deutscher's (2003, p. 19) questions on colonialism and Derridean hospitality, I suggest that it is important to rethink what psychology does to refugees in the name of humanitarian compassion. Having explored the role of confession, doesn't the language of psychology fortify the idea that the dispossessed as guests are lacking something that the host, in the role of the master has? 'In fact, doesn't it reinforce a myth in which the master is highly invested?' (Deutscher, 2003, p. 19). Invested in the sense that acquires a form of language which besides a passage, promises physical and legal occupation in his own territory. The western psychological language as it performs in the landscape of 'emotional hospitality' it claims both compassion and status, aspiring to a homogenous, self-identical and united expression of suffering. However, the language of suffering is culture in disguise. Post-colonial thinkers have well-established the connection between language and culture (Spivak, 1988).

Derrida in the *Monolingualism of the Other* (as cited in Deutscher, 2003, p. 11) has indicated that hospitality is also a form of culture and culture may be itself colonial. What if, therefore, the expression of suffering in this monolingual perspective reflects a form of culture itself? What if emotional hospitality is a form of culture which is inherently colonial? Or to put it in Deutscher's words, 'what if colonialism is the condition of hospitality' and thus emotional hospitality initiates its guests in its own mono-psycho-lingual perspective? Then, as unlikely as it may seem, it is crucial to put forward a general working hypothesis that will not only attempt to situate the provision of psychosocial support to refugees in the inter-governmental 'emotional hospitality' or the way Ψ as method work as monolingual expression of what constitutes *life* for them, but it will also explore the ways under which emotional hospitality is simultaneously constructed and deconstructed.

As Caputo (Derrida & Caputo, 1997; as cited in Nayak, 2015, p. 108) explains: ' Derrida's interest in exploring the tensions within 'hospitality' is not aimed at cynically unmasking it as just more mastery and power ... hospitality is inhabited from within, inwardly disturbed by these tensions, but he does this precisely in order to open hospitality up, to keep it on guard against itself, on the qui vive, to open – to push – it beyond itself. For it is only that internal tension and instability that keeps the idea of hospitality alive, open loose.' Hence, psychology as method besides a conceptual and methodological tool, it is above all a question of politics. A question of politics about the way in which forms of compassion and subjectivity, forms of confession and conversion, are constructed and deconstructed amid psycho-therapeutic discourses of compassion. In Mezzadra and Neilson's words (Mezzadra & Neilson, 2012, p. 66) 'it is above all a question of politics, about the kinds of social worlds and subjectivities produced at the border and the way our work plays into and intervenes in these practices'. For them, border is a site of struggle.

Taking into consideration that borders are not only physical but also relational, it is inevitable to ask what the language of psychology does to refugees and how do refugees resist in this psychological discourse or how do they re-invent it. Nayak (2015) in her book *Race, Gender and the Activism of Black Feminist Theory: Working with Audre Lorde*, makes such a re-invention of the psyche borders by asking us to be 'in the borderland of the self'. The term 'borderland' is coming from Anzaldúa (1987) and is a process of personal and social identity construction and reconstruction that tackles control, domination, oppression. Borrowing the latter term, Nayak (2015, p. 115) argues that 'Being in the "borderland" of self involves giving up inherited inhabitance of the habit of border'. Psychology and humanitarian compassion constitute the psyche borders in which we come to understand both ourselves and the Other(s). Giving them up would mean to reconstitute the borderland of our-selves with the Other and let a dialectic of class, race, gender and struggle begin. It may be there that dignity lies while guests and hosts identities start to become loose and elusive.

Conclusion

If humanitarian compassion and psychology constitute two of the tools that the host acquires, can they ever dismantle his house? Rethinking the latter in what Lorde (1979/1984, p. 112) said '*the master's tools will never dismantle the master's house*' humanitarian compassion, psychology and salvation can only provisionally reconstitute a sense of freedom.

Are these our only tools?

Notes

1. I use the word 'victim' to highlight how the humanitarian discourse represent people amid these circumstances.
2. Ψ as method has been inspired by and is situated within the work of Kapsali and Mentinis (2020) on Trauma as Method, Burman (2019) on *Fanon, Education, Action: Child as Method*, Siddiqui's (2017) elaboration on 'Ghost as Method', Mezzadra and Neilson (2013) on *Border as Method* and Chen (2010) on *Asia as Method: Towards Deimperialization.*
3. The latter does not mean neither that refugees are powerless not that they do not resist. During my work and field study, I came across protests outside of the hotspots and camps, demonstrations inside hotspots and camps, hunger strikes, feminist solidarity, LGBTQI+ solidarity networks among others. Also, refugees use the language of psychology to take some documents that they may help them with their asylum application.

Disclosure statement

No potential conflict of interest was reported by the author.

References

Anzaldúa, G. (1987). *Borderlands. La Frontera: The New Mestiza*. Aunt Lute Books.

Barnett, M. (2011). *Empire of humanity: A history of humanitarianism*. Cornell University Press.

Bistoen, G. (2016). *Trauma, ethics and the political beyond PTSD*. Palgrave Macmillan.

Burman, E. (2019). *Fanon, education, action: Child as method*. Brunner-Routledge.

Chen, K. H. (2010). *Asia as method: Toward deimperialization*. Duke University Press.

Derrida, J. (1999). *Autour de Jacques Derrida: Manifeste pour l'hospitalite*. Paroles de l'aube.

Derrida, J. (2000). *Of hospitality: Anne Dufourmantelle invites Jacques Derrida to respond* (R. Bowlby, Trans.). Stanford University Press.

Derrida, J. (2003). Hostipitality. *Angelaki: Journal of the Theoretical Humanities*, *5*(3), 3–18. https://doi.org/10.1080/09697250020034706

Derrida, J., & Caputo, J. D. (1997). *Deconstruction in a Nutshell: A conversation with Jacques Derrida* (J. D. Caputo, Ed.). Fordham University Press.

Deutscher, P. (2003). Already lamenting: Deconstruction, immigration, colonialism. *Studies in Practical Philosophy*, *3*(1), 5–21. https://doi.org/10.5840/studpracphil2003313

De Vos, J. (2011). The psychologisation of humanitarian aid: Skimming the battlefield and the disaster zone. *History of the Human Sciences*, *24*(3), 103–122. https://doi.org/10.1177/0952695111398572

Fassin, D. (2007). Humanitarianism as a politics of life. *Public Culture*, *19*(3), 499–520. https://doi.org/10.1215/08992363-2007-007

Foucault, M. (1976/1978). *The history of sexuality. Volume I: An introduction* (R. Hurley, Ed.). Pantheon Books.

Goodman, S., Sirriyeh, A., & McMahon, S. (2017). The evolving (Re)categorisations of refugees throughout the 'refugee/migrant crisis'. *Journal of Community & Applied Social Psychology*, *27*(2), 105–114. https://doi.org/10.1002/casp.2302

Kapsali, A., & Mentinis, M. (2018). *Ψυχολογίες Συμμόρφωσης: Σημειώσεις πάνω στον Ψυχοπολιτικό Έλεγχο του Μεταναστευτικού* [Psychologies of compliance: Notes on the psychopolitical control of migration] (in Greek). Oposito.

Kapsali, A., & Mentinis, M. (2020). Το τραύμα ως μέθοδος: Η περίπτωση της Ν. [Trauma as Method: The case of N.]. *Misfit*, *1*, 43–54.

Khiabany, G. (2016). Refugee crisis, imperialism, and pitiless wars on the poor. *Media, Culture & Society*, *38*(5), 755–762. https://doi.org/10.1177/0163443716655093

Lorde, A. (1979/1984). The master's tools will never dismantle the mater's house. In A. Lorde (Ed.), *Sister outsider: Essays and speeches* (pp. 110–113). The Crossing Press.

Marquer, C., Barry, C., Mouchenik, Y., Hustache, S., Dijibo, D. M., Manzo, M. L., Falissard, B., Révah-Lévy, A., Grais, R. F., & Moro, M. R. (2012). A rapid screening tool for psychological distress in children 3-6 years old: Results of a validation study. *BMC Psychiatry*, *12*(170). https://doi.org/10.1186/1471-244X-12-170

Mezzadra, S., & Neilson, B. (2012). Between inclusion and exclusion: On the topology of global space and borders. *Theory, Culture & Society*, *29*(4/5), 58–75. https://doi.org/10.1177/0263276412443569

Mezzadra, S., & Neilson, B. (2013). *Border as method.* Duke University Press.

Mills, C. (2013). *Decolonizing global mental health. The psychiatrization of the majority world.* Routledge.

Mohanty, C. T. (1984). Under western eyes: Feminist scholarship and colonial discourses. *Boundary 2*, *12*(3), 333–358. https://doi.org/10.2307/302821

Nayak, S. (2015). *Race, gender and the activism of black feminist theory: Working with Audre Lorde.* Routledge.

Oliver, K. (2017). Earthquakes: Deconstructing humanitarianism. *Derrida Today*, *10*(1), 38–50. https://doi.org/10.3366/drt.2017.0141

Parker, I. (2007). *Revolution in psychology: Alienation to emancipation.* Pluto Press.

Pupavac, V. (2004). Psychosocial interventions and the demoralisation of humanitarianism. *Journal of Biosocial Science*, *36*(4), 491–504. https://doi.org/10.1017/S0021932004006613

Redfield, P., & Bornstein, E. (2010). An Introduction to the anthropology of humanitarianism. In E. Bornstein & P. Redfield (Eds.), *Forces of compassion: Humanitarianism between ethics and politics* (pp. 3–30). School for Advanced Research Press.

Siddiqui, S. (2017, August 21–25). A turn to ghost in social science theorising. In *Presentation at the International Society for Theoretical Psychology Conference.* Rikkyo University.

Spivak, G. C. (1988). Can the subaltern speak? In C. Nelson & L. Grossberg (Eds.), *Marxism and the interpretation of culture* (pp. 267–310). University of Illinois Press .

Summerfield, D. (1997). Legacy of war: Beyond "Trauma" to the social fabric. *The Lancet*, *349*, 1568. https://doi.org/10.1016/S0140-6736(05)61627-3

Summerfield, D. (1999). A critique of seven assumptions behind psychological trauma programmes in war-affected areas. *Social Science & Medicine*, *48*(10), 1449–1462. https://doi.org/10.1016/S0277-9536(98)00450-X

Vaughn, M. (1991). *Curing their ills. Colonial power and African illness.* Stanford University Press.

Diversity and aggression: A reflection on sensual meanings and an ameliorative law after Freud and Lacan

Tony McSherry

ABSTRACT
The aim of this article is to explore phenomenologically how the 'inside' (psychical) and 'outside' (the other and/or society) interweave since it appears that sometimes those of us who favour diversity may also inadvertently shut it down. Phenomenology appears to open more easily onto what we don't want to know about in our everyday lives, or a turning away which impedes diversity. If we cannot hear our own thoughts that come to us from the 'inside', then how can we move towards diversity on the 'outside'. The tensions between turning away and turning towards leads into a Freudian look at conscience and aggression, and Lacan's idea of the ego being the seat of identification and misrecognition. Freud's observation of an 'original' aggression towards the other appears especially important. It is argued that this aggression always fragments the movement towards diversity. Two factors appear to mediate this movement, namely a 'negative' exclusion, and a 'positive' ameliorative 'law'. Two fictional accounts are given from everyday life reflecting societal and psychical aggression, including its 'privacy' or sensual meanings.

Phenomenology, Freud, and speaking for yourself

Most of us would agree that questions of diversity bring up questions of morality and ethics. And this then brings us into the field of 'conscience'. A number of ideas present themselves like shadows immediately here: What is it that 'I' think (or what is it that 'you' think, reader) about diversity? Is diversity about 'loving your neighbour as yourself'? Is diversity a good thing? And almost like an unwelcome stranger, the word 'aggression' moves like a cold current amongst my thoughts. 'I' is in inverted commas because the 'I' is what has to take seriously these experiences of cold currents, shadows, and unexpected arrivals in the psyche when we talk of ourselves as if we were coherent wholes. At the risk of being moralistic, we must take these experiences seriously at least if we are serious about being therapists, and not just moralists. The 'I' here was originally intended as a phenomenological I, that which is not 'you', but it also brings to mind the 'I' of Freud's (1933/1964, p. 80) ethical aim of analysis as '*Wo es war, soll Ich werden*' - ('where it was, shall I be'), and this is a real movement that comes from being with others who are interested and make space for that 'I' and that 'it'. My own thoughts here are that whatever the 'I' is, it is more about something that is largely unknown, although there are many who live in the certainty that this is not the case.

In *The Ethics of Psychoanalysis: The Seminar of Jacques Lacan Book VII* (2008/1986, p. 8), Lacan encourages the reader to read again 'an indispensable work', *Civilisation and Its Discontents* (Freud, 1933/1964), 'unsurpassed for an understanding of Freud's thought and the summation of his experience'. Both Freud and Lacan are speaking about everyday life, and the bizarre achievements that involve us living together with such conflicting interests at all. Clearly, things break down, and are recovered sometimes. It is difficult to begin even to speak of one's own experience of everyday life, and at least in my case I needed 'permission' from others, and others to 'light the way' until I found my own voice to throw its own light. Voices illuminate. My guiding lights now are the phenomenologists such as Husserl and Merleau-Ponty and others, along with colleagues, therapists, clients, and friends, and also the psychoanalysts, especially Freud and Lacan, but also others.

Phenomenology is to say what is there, what is shown in our experience in all its intricate and sensual detail - 'original self-evidences. . . and every other manner of intuition' (Husserl, 1970; §34 cited in Welton, 1999, p. 367). This is not to say that such experiences are 'facts', but they tell us something about ourselves and the other.

Experience goes beyond the given meanings of the words we find to describe that experience and into the realm of the sensual or private meanings of a language that emerges from that experience (see McSherry et al., 2019). In an attempt to say what is there, there is what Husserl calls the reduction (epoché), a 'leading back' to what he was hoping were the structures of consciousness.

> . . . through the epoché a new way of experiencing, of thinking, of theorizing, is opened to the philosopher; here, situated *above* his own natural being and *above* the natural world, he loses nothing of their being and their objective truths. (Husserl, 1970, p. 152; cited in Zahavi, 2003, p. 45 original italics)

I find in Freud a parallel here, in that 'psychoanalysis' is like a leading back to something quite simple and what then gets called a theory by those who do not accept that it is a journey; through dreams, ideas about recurring patterns, deepening insights, analyses, and revisions. It is the journey that one makes to such simplicity that involves the difficult and sometimes beautiful landscapes of the sensual, those experiences of the privacy of the mind that can perhaps only be spoken of in therapy, or in a dialogue of the soul to itself, and can rarely be offered up to the understandings of 'given' meanings; those meanings 'given' like things we find in dictionaries or theories that circulate in solid, sedimented forms, that are necessary for everyday communication but kill off the living breath of understanding; 'given' meanings that also form the impositions of ethical and moral codes in organisations and society. The 'sensual' or private meanings we find ourselves subject to are not always in line with the 'given' meanings we also find circulating in the psyche, and the interaction between the two surely has something to do with the activity of conscience.

It is in the attempt to 'lead back' away from our assumptions, impositions, and interpolations, that we discover ourselves and what we do to the other, whilst at the same time making room for the other and what the other does to us. This 'leading back' is one way to think of how you discover your sensual relation to the world (of others, of memory, of time, of being embodied), of how we are forever entangled in it and can never 'get outside' it fully. It takes courage to confront this entanglement, and not the kind of 'dead' courage of the 'objective' scientist (or moralist) in the service of some ridiculous goal of objectivity - who can put aside her theories in the face of new 'data' - but rather the living courage to face that one's life perhaps has been all a journey to ruin, or a castle built on sand, or that one's very psyche has been a violent attack on others (for example).

Lacan's encouragement to read *Civilisation and Discontents*, and Freud's thoughts on conscience, I took personally, especially the following:

> And here at last an idea comes in that belongs entirely to psychoanalysis, and is foreign to our ordinary way of thinking . . . For it tells us that although at first it is conscience (or, rather, the fear that later becomes the conscience) that causes us to renounce the drives, this causal relation is later reversed. *Every renunciation of the drives now becomes a dynamic source of conscience*; every fresh renunciation reinforces its severity and intolerance . . . which then demands further renunciation. (Freud, 1933/1964, p. 94 italics added)

He clarifies using the example of aggression:

> A considerable measure of aggressivity must have developed in the child against the authority that deprives him of his first (and most significant) satisfactions, no matter what kinds of deprivations were required. The child is obliged to forgo the satisfaction of this vengeful aggression . . . By means of identification he incorporates this unassailable authority into himself; it now becomes the super-ego . . . however, the original severity of the super-ego is not . . . the severity that one has experienced from him [the father] or attributes to him; *it represents rather one's own aggression towards him.* (Freud, 1933/1964, p. 96 italics added)

Lacan (2008, p. 239) summarises,

> . . . at the heart of everything Freud taught, one finds the following: the energy of the so-called superego derives from the aggression the subject turns back upon himself.

Why are these observations about aggression important regarding diversity? I will try to answer this giving two accounts. Both are works of fiction aimed at highlighting some of the fraught ambivalence of experience in terms of diversity and thoughts that we find ourselves thinking. Whilst this may open the door to committing a kind of solipsistic idealism, I argue that we are always embedded in the world. Even in a psychotic state the person draws on the world – so that even delusions reflect the world as it presents itself, however distorted. People did not involve Martians in delusional states until such ideas were already circulating through science (telescopes) and fiction (novels). Just as the mind is embodied so too is the body 'en-minded' (to coin a phrase). Each is dissolved in the other.

A fictional and imaginary phenomenology

A takeaway. A Saturday evening darkness descending. Why I'm here is another story. It is not my usual place to have dinner and it brings fleeting rose-tinted memories of being a very young man caught in relationships and hopes that seemed simple. And there is something about the bright lights, the clean white tables, the clean glass separating the cold of the outside from the warmth of the inside that makes me feel safe, and fleeting other worlds shine and glimmer, fragmented memories catching the light like the reflections on the huge glass window panes as if not knowing anymore who is inside or outside, what is real or imagined. You can get your order at your table these days and I wait patiently, my attention flicking from my phone on the news about Ukraine to the other tables. Close by a family of four children and their father. The youngest, a girl, about 4, presses her father unselfconsciously for more, for different things her siblings have, pulling his arm and climbing on him if they do not comply. The eldest, about 11, is a girl trying to define her own space at the table, using her arms to frame it, to keep her little brother and sister from stealing her food, glancing around in embarrassment at the noise they make. Her little brother especially seems intent on getting her attention, and he is only happy when she punches him on the thigh and he squeals with delight. The punch is soft and with the flat of her fist not her knuckles. The fourth child, a girl about a year younger than the eldest, sits almost shining and solemn-eyed – it seems naturally, aloof from the rest – and her father goes to get a carton of milk for her when she asks. When he leaves, the two youngest immediately pounce on the eldest and she responds patiently, no punches. I imagine she is behaving like her mother would and I am suddenly aware she is aware I am looking at her. I smile slightly at her and hope she will understand that with the benevolence intended. It is almost impossible nowadays to smile at or be benevolent towards a child without there being some monstrous possibility in the air – perhaps rightly so. I catch her father's eye as he returns with the milk, to dispel that. He is about 25 years younger than me, and is quite beautiful. No wedding ring. He seemed harassed by and protective of his children. His look makes me think he is from the Levant somewhere, and his children make me think their mother is white British and is also beautiful. A polite teenager finds my table with my order. Is it a dinner, or a meal? It is something to eat, I suppose, and it seems quite good enough. They have run out of carrot sticks so she put in apple slices instead. Smiles and thanks. She is gone before I notice there is no milk with the tea. I am reading Kavanagh (1964/1972) in school in 1979.

Then as a teenager filled with anxiety about growing up, and apprehension and optimism, I felt what it meant. Some glittering luxurious fabric of being that only a child could notice properly. But that only a child is exposed to, and can suffer through also. Kavanagh was a favourite of our old English teacher who died that year. I can still hear his gravelly voice, a stream polishing sentences, the chalk scraping on slate. It's important to get the tea bag out quickly or the tea gets too strong. The cardboard wrapping on the wrap is a struggle. How are you meant to eat it?

The family have left. Their table is pristine, with one tray piled high neatly with the wrappings and leftovers. I miss them, and realise that I feel lonely. In a few seconds I imagine the lives they will live. Apart from the ordinary horrors of everyday living, will they have to go through racism and bias as they grow up?

There is a kind of movement to my right – a group of about twelve young teenagers. They take up three tables adjacent to each other and nearby. Closest to me is a tall black girl – Do I call her black, or is that wrong? She is arguing playfully with a thin, smaller boy. Something about a portable phone charger, and he snatches it from her and she laughs. He laughs too. There is a flow of affection between them and I recall what the phenomenologists mean by intentionality, that our consciousness is always towards something and in a certain way. Something flowing between people. His hair is styled and his clothes are a pale blue matching track suit and matching trainers. Her hair is styled too, braided and tied back, and her clothes are denim jeans and a white top. She has white trainers. They mirror the whole group, teenagers in different coloured clothes but in style and rapport similar dress and presentation. Their 'at ease-ness' with each other is striking. And striking too is what happens when one of them has to leave. One has to be home by 8, and his friend says to wait that he will walk to the bus stop too. As they stand the whole group stand in twos and threes, and everyone takes turns to hug those who are leaving. There is smiling and talk, as if long-lost friends are meeting and saying goodbye. Yet it is more like a ritual of bonding, care, and intimacy. Perhaps I am idealising it. I don't stare, and turn to my book on Machiavelli, reading the thoughts of a beautiful mind between bites of the chicken wrap.

> For a long time I have not said what I believed, nor do I ever believe what I say. And if sometimes I do happen to tell the truth, I hide it among so many lies that it is hard to find. (Machiavelli, 1521/2018 in Benner, 2018, p. xviii)

I notice that I am invisible to the group, too old, too undefined now to be of importance. They look through me like I am part of the mirage on the window glass. One of the bigger boys looks through that glass - 'God there's loads of them' - and I can discern across the street a group of darkly dressed figures moving with a mutinous energy.

They soon cross the road and have flowed into the spaces between the tables like a group of jostling wild creatures, but in their uniform of black track suits and black trainers. They seem to be looking for someone. About eight of these boys sit around a central table, and one or two keep standing. In their forefront is a small boy with a loud voice, shouting and as if speaking for them all, 'Who's looking at me? Are you looking at me?' He is only addressing his peers in the place; at first a group of four meek-looking boys queuing. Their meekness incites him and he shouts, 'I'll have you when you get outside' but they look away. He then turns his attention to the bigger boy in the colourful group, and repeats his challenge. The bigger boy does not respond in kind, but neither does he turn away. Instead, he waits and when the small boy repeats himself he asks has he done anything wrong to him. In the split second of silence that follows, a slight opening of a pause in which to think, nobody seems to think in the black-clad group until a girl intervenes. She is from the black-clad group – wearing a black suit, not a track suit, with another girl dressed the same – and she says to the aggressive boy, 'We know them. They live near us'. The girl's intervention breaks the tension, and the two boys pump fists. Something dissolves. The small boy remains talking at the table as the rest of his group move outside. The girls seem to be almost parental now, and his aggressive façade drops for a moment and then returns. I imagine he needs a father to show him the way, to assuage some angst in his psyche. It is not a mother he needs, I hear myself speaking to myself. I don't know why. Perhaps I am speaking for my own anxious teenage self. His group are messing about outside, shouting along with sounds of a bin being kicked. He follows the noise outside. High spirits.

When I look up next, most of the colourful group have started to leave. There are hugs and a lot of talking. This showing of affection and loyalty amongst young teenagers is moving and somehow mesmerising. There is some activity of the psyche happening here that seemed to contrast so sharply with the dark-clad group. I imagined there was some ameliorative force at work, some discourse of the mind in play for the colour-clad group, so that potential aggressions and rivalries could be resolved by speaking, touch, affection, forming some common bond. Perhaps I wished this to be so. It seemed undeveloped in the dark-clad group apart from the calming intervention of the girl. And it showed itself in the bigger boy's appeal to a dialogue with the small boy rather than an attack of some kind. But the black-suited girls had left now, and the boys took up places across two tables in the corner near the door. Three of the colour-clad group remained, all girls. They were on their phones a lot, texting. One bought an ice cream. One of the dark-clad boys, tall and thin, kept coming over to them. He sat skew-ways at their table, and pointed a poking finger at the prettiest one, demanding an answer to 'Hey you! Yeah, you. Who are you?' The girl glanced up, mumbled something, and went back to her phone. Perhaps it was the safety of the place, the presence of adults around, the security cameras, and their phones, that made them seem unperturbed. Even so, the girls were far less confident and talkative now that the rest of their group had left. He went back to his group. A plastic bottle of juice flew past the girls and crashed into a chair nearby. Some adults looked up. The cleaner told the boys off and they laughed. The tall boy came back, with the same chat-up line, and the same pointing finger. I went to get some tea and as I passed his chair I felt this urge to kick it from under him. Something primeval that was immediately thought better of by something more reasoned. There would be something awful in such 'following through' in any case, as if some code would be broken that would ruin any outcome. And the girls were in fact safe. But in a different environment they might not be

I returned to my place with the tea, with milk now. Machiavelli's words could reflect how Freud and Lacan in their different ways describe the obfuscations of the ego (whatever says 'I'), constantly at work to hide other feelings, desires and motivations. I think that diversity is a good thing, of course – But it is like an ideal that we can aspire towards, much like we aspire towards something which we are also in denial about, something covered over and lost in a sea of idealistic wishing, social commands, and reversals. Why do I wish to exclude and not try to understand the tall boy at that moment even though it is a moment that will not last? It has something to do with my own abhorrence of violence towards girls and women of course. Perhaps I am misjudging his 'chat up' style? We are not transparent to ourselves. If we were, what kinds of masters of ourselves would this make us? We need others to know ourselves.

Thinking of my takeaway hour or so, I have been in proximity to a young family, where clearly the protection and safety was coming from the father, and then also surrounded by groups of young teenagers, where the sense of protection and safety was coming from an instilment of some similar psychical authority. Such an authority seemed to me to be more fragile in the dark-clad group (the need for the 'uniform' perhaps indicating this?). One group portrays dialogue, care, sensuality, sexuality, ameliorated aggression, the overflowing energy of youth. The other all of these too, but perhaps more dominated by a less ameliorated aggression.

A dream and a mediator

Outward-directed aggression can be directed inwards also of course. Aggression shows itself in the attack upon oneself. And this is my second much briefer account. Once on waking from a garbled dream, there was left around me like a swamp a deep feeling of being 'no good' - of being 'emptied out' of value. As if it is an attack on the self by the self. Or as if I have wandered into a bottomless swamp somewhere in the landscape of the psyche. This is what Freud means by conscience generating renunciation and the renunciation generating conscience – there is an aggression directed at the self which could have no limit. The monstrous superego demands more and more. That is, in the absence of something ameliorative. I suppose that in that absence, no wonder the smaller boy might have to 'get rid of it' somewhere – finding it in another who was 'looking at him'. In the clamour for diversity then (accept me, recognise me, and acknowledge my knowledge of myself), I find my own aggression towards the other, that butts up against the limits of my own self. These limits are not necessarily permanent. This is an aggression that seems to know no limits unless a limit has already been instilled or found solid ground in oneself. And it seems we don't know our limits until we find them through others.

One of the first people I remember as being therapeutic said that he had time to 'walk alongside' me. He would light a small candle on the table by us and somehow a space would open up. I was like a rag-and-bone dealer emptying my soul of its shabby contents, but his interest would make those shameful things shine as if they were port keys to fantastic places. And they were. Like lights shining into old tombs, or new suns rising on new worlds. The aggression directed at the self from the self is ameliorated by a person, and finds a ground – a limit to the aggression – that was already there. A diversity of the psyche is coming into being here. The more we accept and understand our own entanglements, the more we are able to try to accept and understand those of others. If you try to pin it down you will lose the magic of its 'privacy' however, and collapse everything into socially agreed 'given' meanings.

Lacan (2008, p. 239) says it is the steadying hand of the Law – one that is instilled in the psyche somehow – that ameliorates, that imposes a limit, a 'mediation' on the superego. This law is not the old patriarchal archaic one of 'Love thy neighbour as thyself' - because if we love ourselves with such condemning, righteous aggression (think of the dream) that leads us only towards such aggression – but rather an ameliorating love that comes from outside, elsewhere (see Lacan, 2008, pp. 238–239).

An ameliorative law

In trying to understand what kind of law is this that 'ameliorates', I am drawn to the older boy who opted for dialogue, and also to the suited girl who opted for inclusion. And the older girl in the family who became the 'mother' when the father left momentarily. And also my 'first therapist'. I also think of Zizek's thoughts on St Paul's love with his Lacanian twist emptying it of its religious content.

> In other words, the point of the claim that even if I were to possess all knowledge, without love, I would be nothing, is not simply that *with* love, I am 'something' - in love, *I am also nothing* but, as it were, a Nothing humbly aware of itself, A Nothing paradoxically made rich through the very awareness of its lack. Only a lacking, vulnerable being is capable of love: the ultimate mystery of love then is therefore that incompleteness is in a way *higher than completion.* On the one hand, only an imperfect, lacking being loves: we love because we do *not* know all. (Žižek, 2000, p. 147 original italics)

When we speak of diversity then, who do we include? I include the young family, and the colour-clad group without thinking, but some elements in my psyche are baulking at some members of the dark-clad group for reasons we cannot speak of here although I still want to make room for them. All of these 'decisions' have private, or 'sensual' meanings, that cannot be discussed fully on the page, and to tear them apart into the language of socially prescribed – 'public' - norms ('given' meanings) can be a violence. And herein lies an ethical role for psychotherapy and counselling with respect to questions of diversity: it provides a space for the sensual meanings of a person's world to come into contact with given meanings, but without retribution or condemnation. My therapist by candle-light was not a qualified therapist at all, yet he provided a space that allowed something private to find a voice. A not so far cry from that candle light, in the stark dream lights of a takeaway the fictional characters are perhaps all *within us* to some extent. How we react to them, including the narrator, at a visceral level is what we need to understand.

A conclusion

Diversity is a good thing. And the characters bow out now: the isolated older person, invisible to a society obsessed with youth, and youth obsessed with itself; the vulnerable teenage girls always so close to potential male violence; the cleaner being laughed at; meek boys filled with fear; a divorced father with nowhere else to take his children; vulnerable boys with no sense of belonging apart from the clothes they wear. As a simple thought experiment, imagine the narrator here as a teenage boy, and the two groups adults – How different would our thoughts be on him being in this situation? Views are multiple and diverse.

But what Freud discovered is still so important – and especially with respect to diversity – because we repress what we do not want to know about... But that doesn't mean that what we have repressed is our 'true self'. The problem is that we have to repress something in order to live amongst others, because society makes it so, and we often repress it (and others who remind us of it) with the utmost aggression. The societal forces that advocate for diversity too are perhaps the same. They want to take their place with the powerful, righteous 'superego'. Perhaps that is the way they have to be in order to be heard, but something is always in danger of being excluded in the process. So the question about how to achieve diversity may instead be better served if we ask, 'What will we agree on that we can exclude (for now)?' and think about that carefully.

It also seems important to appreciate 'righteous' aggression but without falling into the trap of thinking that it is always benevolent. Ask yourself what you will do when you have achieved diversity: Will you enclose it? Will only certain others be allowed in to the enclosure? People who think like you? If we are really honest the answer to that question could well be a 'yes'.

Tony McSherry is an Existential-Analytical psychotherapist (UKCP – SAFPAC/CEC) working in private practice. He has special interests in phenomenology, existentialism and psychoanalysis, and is critical of scientism in the therapies. He is a member of the Critical Psychotherapy Network. In his PhD work he investigated the nature of the therapeutic relationship in mental health nursing and what it is that is therapeutic in relationships. He is currently working on a phenomenology of being a psychotherapist.

Disclosure statement

No potential conflict of interest was reported by the author.

References

Benner, E. (2018). *Be like the fox: Machiavelli's lifelong quest for freedom*. Penguin Books.

Freud, S. (1930/2014). *Civilisation and its discontents* (D. McClintock, Trans.). Penguin Classics.

Freud, S. (1933/1964). New introductory lectures on psychoanalysis. In J. Strachey (Ed.), *The standard edition of the complete psychological works of Sigmund Freud* (Vol. XXII, pp. 1–182). Hogarth Press.

Husserl, E. (1970). *The crisis of European sciences and transcendental phenomenology: An introduction to phenomenological philosophy* (D. Carr, Trans.). Northwestern University Press.

Kavanagh, P. (1964/1972). Advent. In *Collected poems* (p. 70). Martin Brian & O'Keefe Ltd.

Lacan, J. (2008). *The ethics of psychoanalysis: The seminar of Jacques Lacan Book VII.* Routledge.

Machiavelli, N. (1521/2018). *Letter to Gucciardini.*

McSherry, T., Loewenthal, D., & Cayne, J. (2019). A phenomenology of the therapeutic after Husserl and Merleau-Ponty. *Existential analysis (30.1) 30th anniversary Pearl edition*, 128–143.

Welton, D. (1999). *The essential Husserl: Basic writings in transcendental phenomenology.* Indiana University Press.

Zahavi, D. (2003). *Husserl's phenomenology.* Stanford University Press.

Žižek, S. (2000). *The Fragile absolute – or, why is the Christian legacy worth fighting for?.* Verso.

An exploration of lesbian and gay people's experiences of religion, and their implications for psychotherapy: An Interpretative Phenomenological Analysis (IPA)

Peter Meades

ABSTRACT

This qualitative research uses Interpretive Phenomenological Analysis (IPA) to explore lesbian and gay people's experiences of Christianity, Islam, and Judaism, and the implications for psychotherapy. A total of six participants, three gay men and three lesbian women, were identified through an initial online survey and successive purposive sampling. Data were collected using unstructured interviews and analysed to determine three major themes: 'Religious Tribalism', 'Liminal Processes', and 'Navigating Relationships'. In the context of a wider social discourse regarding heterosexist hegemony, this project has the potential to increase psychotherapists' awareness of the intersection of homosexuality and religion, and the diverse ways in which this plays out. The research invites therapists to consider any potentially socially constructed positions, and encourages a life-course perspective. Recommendations include providing high-quality training for therapists to understand, appreciate and interact with people from different cultures or belief systems from their own. Suggestions for future research include exploring heterosexual perspectives from within religious institutions, and exploration of the positive role of religion for non-heterosexual people.

1. Introduction

There have undoubtedly been significant improvements for gender, sexual and relationship diversities (GSRD), but it is argued there is still widespread intolerance of same-sex attraction and non-binary gender identities (Davies, 2007). Reinforcing this point is the fact that homosexuality is illegal in seventy-four countries of the world, and the death penalty is still active in ten.

The main aim of this research is to explore six lesbian and gay people's experiences of Christianity, Islam and Judaism, to consider the findings in relation to the wider literature, and consider their implications on the field of psychotherapy.

2. Literature review

Historically, pathological notions of human sexuality have combined with powerful prevailing religious attitudes to intensify socio-political censure and control according to Bowers et al. (2010). Therefore, religion and homosexual orientation were considered incongruous. The dominant religions often appear to be so powerfully anti-gay that, for gay and lesbian people, choosing to stay within an institution feels tantamount to 'sleeping with the enemy' (Yip, 2010a, p. 42).

According to Bowers et al. (2010), psychotherapists may inadvertently get caught between a positive, affirmative healthy lifestyle model, and a culturally rooted, religious-based heterosexist system of attitudes and constraints. This relates to unconscious bias – that we may hold views borne out of socially conservative, religious-based heterosexist constructs, which may not be helpful to clients. Similarly, people can sometimes turn to religion, appealing to a higher power for understanding and support (Bent-Goodley & Fowler, 2006). However, when this place of sanctuary is turned against lesbian and gay people, this can lead to significant mental distress (Super & Jacobson, 2012).

Dubious translations of religious texts across theistic religions have resulted in generations of people whose beliefs and values are unreliably informed (Helminiak, 1994). Authors frequently point to six isolated passages from the Christian Bible, (Genesis, 19: 1–8; Leviticus, 18:22, 20:13; Romans 1:26, 27; 1 Corinthians, 6:9; 1 Timothy 1:10) that are verses that support conservative Christians' contention that homosexuality is a sin (Rodriguez, 2010). Christian doctrine has decreed homosexuality to be 'unnatural', and an 'abomination in the eyes of God' based almost entirely on those six passages (Clarke et al., 1990).

Most religions across the world categorise behaviours associated with homosexuality as 'unnatural', 'ungodly', and 'impure' (Yip, 2005). Melton (1991) found that 72% of Christian religious organizations condemned homosexuality as being 'an abomination'. Research into the tolerance of homosexuality among non-Judeo-Christian groups has, according to Adamczyk and Pitt (2009), been minimal, a fact that they put down to the smaller population of non-Abrahamic religious organisations in the West.

Coyle and Rafalin (2000) point out that the Torah is widely believed to be clear in its prohibition of sexual activity between men, and by extension, male homosexuality. They acknowledge there are significant divergences between the expectations of men and women within Judaism. In the case of men, the failure to marry and produce an heir can often be viewed as a type of 'communal treason' (Unterman, 1995, p. 68).

The severe penalties, including death, for people found guilty of 'homosexual immorality' in many Muslim countries, suggests that religious authorities are more likely to interpret religious doctrine as prohibiting homosexuality (Helie, 2004). Adamczyk and Pitt (2009) argue that, where the religious context is more disapproving in Muslim nations, anti-gay sentiment is disseminated throughout public discourse, public institutions, legal codes, social norms, and family structures.

King et al. (2008) conducted a systematic review and meta-analysis of the prevalence of mental disorder, substance misuse, suicide, suicidal ideation, and deliberate self-harm in LGB people and confirmed that LGB people are at higher risk than heterosexual people. Bachmann and Gooch (2018) surveyed 5000 LGBT people in the UK on behalf of Stonewall and found that 52% of participants experienced depression in the previous year, 13% had attempted to take their own life, 46% had thought about taking their life, 16% said they had drunk alcohol every day over the previous year, 13% had taken drugs at least once a month over the previous year, 23% had witnessed discriminatory remarks by healthcare staff, 5% had been pressured to access services to question or change their sexual-orientation when accessing healthcare services, 19% were not out to any healthcare professional about their sexual-orientation when seeking general medical care, and 14% had avoided treatment for fear of discrimination. The report uncovers alarmingly high rates of poor mental health, and challenges experienced by LGBT people accessing services in the UK in 2018.

Internalised homophobia, or internalised heterosexism (Szymanski & Chung, 2003), happens when anti-gay attitudes are retroflected, resulting in devaluation of the self, internal conflict, and low self-esteem (Meyer & Dean, 1998). Intrinsic religiosity, or strong religious affiliation, was shown to be a strong predictor of internalised homophobia in lesbian and gay people (Herek, 1987).

Shallenberger (1996) suggests that one of the most significant events in a lesbian or gay person's spiritual journey, is 'coming out'. Rodriguez (2010) believes this happens when a person becomes more aware of the discrepancies between living a gay lifestyle and remaining actively involved in organised religion. Shallenberger (1996) found the following key themes relating to the process: deep and often difficult self-questioning, growing self-recognition and self-identification in the face of prolific anti-gay biases from a homophobic and heterosexist culture, sudden or measured disclosure to loved ones, and passage into deeper involvement with the LGBT community (Shallenberger, 1996, p. 197).

Das Nair and Butler (2012) helpfully promote the key concept of intersectionality from the perspective of working psychologically with Gender and Sexual diversities. Their academic work examines specific identities and how they intersect, including: gender, race, ethnicity, religion, refugees and asylum seekers, social class, physical health, mental health, disability, age and ageing.

Empowerment is a central theme and empirical research has repeatedly shown that the intersection of sexuality and religion plays out in diverse ways, leading to multiple outcomes (Yip, 2014). This is especially true when framed within a life-course perspective, for example, someone who starts from a position of guilt and shame can learn to transcend and transform, developing spiritual, cultural, and social capital within religious institutions and beyond.

3. Methodology and methods

3.1. Introduction

A qualitative methodology was chosen to achieve a detailed, deep understanding of the topic from the perspective of the participants (Harper & Thompson, 2012). The relational ontological perspective recognises it is not possible to understand reality without considering the context in which the real occurs (Slife, 2004). In seeking to comprehend participants' lived-experiences, I align with an interpretative (hermeneutic) phenomenological epistemology (Larkin & Thompson, 2012). Interpretative Phenomenological Analysis (IPA) has an idiographic focus, offering insights into how a given person, in a given context, makes sense of a given phenomenon (Reid et al., 2005).

3.2. Issues of validity

An initial pilot study was used to test the process. Each interview was transcribed manually, allowing time to dwell with the data, and ensuring there was no outside interference (e.g. computer software).

3.3. Participant sample

A survey method was used to recruit participants. Data were cleaned by applying filters to the total of 345 responses, which resulted in 117 responses, then 57 who agreed to be interviewed. Filters related to inclusion and exclusion criteria (e.g. 'gay', 'lesbian', 'agrees to be contacted for interview'). A further cycle of purposive sampling left 10 participants: 5 gay men, 4 lesbian women, and 1 bisexual woman. Final respondents were emailed, providing initial information about the IPA research project and the interviews. Four participants did not reply, resulting in the final sample of six participants – three gay men and three gay women (Table 1). An information

Table 1. Profile of participants.

Participant Pseudonym	Age Range	Sexual Orientation	Gender Identity	Religion(s) and Branch	Race and Ethnicity
"Rose"	60+	Lesbian	Female	Christianity Catholicism: Roman Catholic	White Irish
"Cate"	21-29	Lesbian	Female	Judaism: Conservative	White Other
"Mark"	50-59	Gay	Male	Christianity Catholicism: Evangelical	White British
"Pam"	60+	Lesbian	Female	Christianity Protestantism: Evangelical	White British
"Paul"	40-49	Gay	Male	Christianity Protestantism: Church of England	White British
"Jay"	30-39	Gay	Male	Islam: Sunni	Asian Pakistani

sheet with consent form was sent to the participants and interviews were arranged.

3.4. Pilot interview

A pilot interview confirmed that unstructured interviews could produce rich data. Recording equipment operated as expected. During the practice pilot interview, the participant's mobile telephone went off and this was experienced as intrusive – a helpful learning point.

3.5. Data collection

Each unstructured interview began with an expansive question, 'So, where would you like to start?' Interviews were recorded using an encrypted digital recorder and were deleted after the interviews were transcribed. Each interview lasted approximately one hour.

3.6. Transcribing interviews

Manual transcribing enabled full immersion. Each interaction on the transcript was coded with a number for reference in the data analysis. Participants' names were replaced with pseudonyms and all identifiers were redacted. Each transcript was read several times before formal data analysis.

3.7. Data analysis

Detailed descriptive and interpretative notes were made on each of the six interview transcripts. Initial noting and emergent themes were developed. This process was repeated. Themes were compared across transcripts with each new transcript being analysed, and from the combined sets of emergent

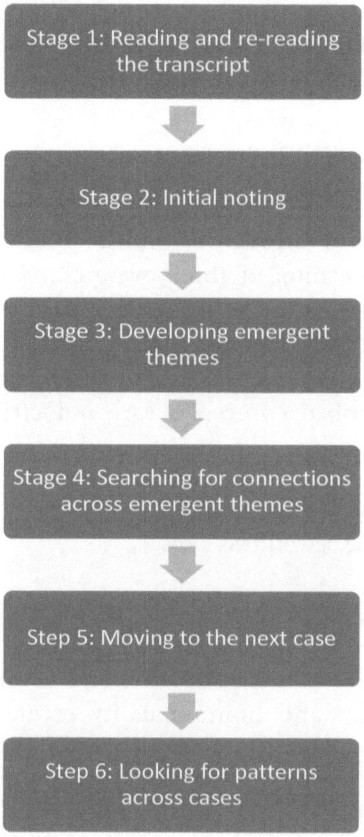

Figure 1. Stages of IPA data analysis.

themes, major themes were developed. After analysing each of the interviews individually, further analysis of the connections continued across interviews, until the final master themes were identified (Figure 1).

3.8. Ethical considerations

Ethical approval was granted by the University Programme Approval Panel. Professional codes of conduct/ethical practice were followed. Data stored on a computer were password protected and encrypted on a memory stick. Transcripts were anonymised and all identifiers removed.

Informed consent to participate was guaranteed by providing a Participant Information Sheet and Consent Form with information about purpose, access to data, data storage, and confidentiality. Participants were advised that professional transcription services would not be used, and the proof reader would receive 'cleaned' write-up.

Wider generalisations were not possible given the idiographic nature of the research and due to the small number of participants (Smith et al., 2009). The author reports no competing interests to declare.

4. Findings and discussion

Themes were interpreted through careful analysis of the interview data resulting in the identification of three overarching master themes represented in Figure 2, along with the related sub-themes that are represented in Figures 3–5. Recurrent themes across participant interviews are shown in Table 2.

All participants described a process of early indoctrination into a religious community:

> It's kind of in your DNA if you've been reared on it . . . I would have been in church regularly at [the age of] two. (Rose)

Yip (2014) points out that for many nonreligious people in secular societies, religion is perceived as a constraining and restrictive force, antithetical to values such as personal liberty, diversity, and pluralism. Therefore, the intersection of religion and homosexuality creates tension, and non-

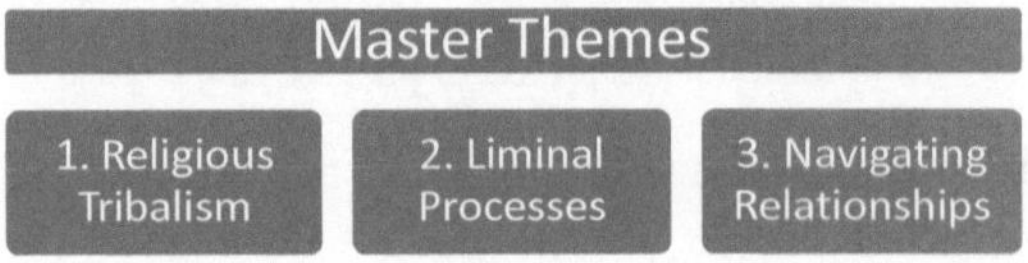

Figure 2. The master themes.

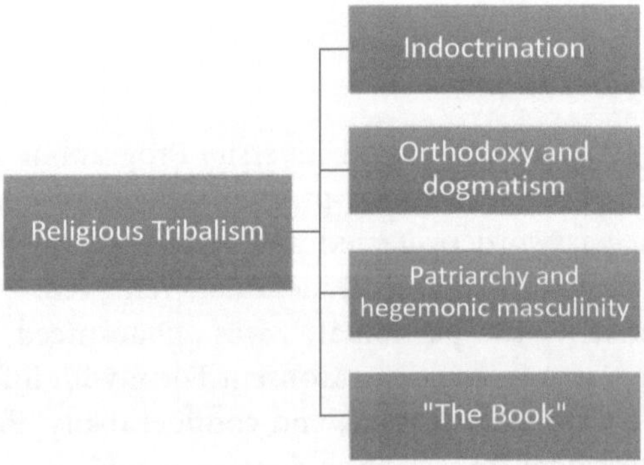

Figure 3. Master theme 1 with sub-themes.

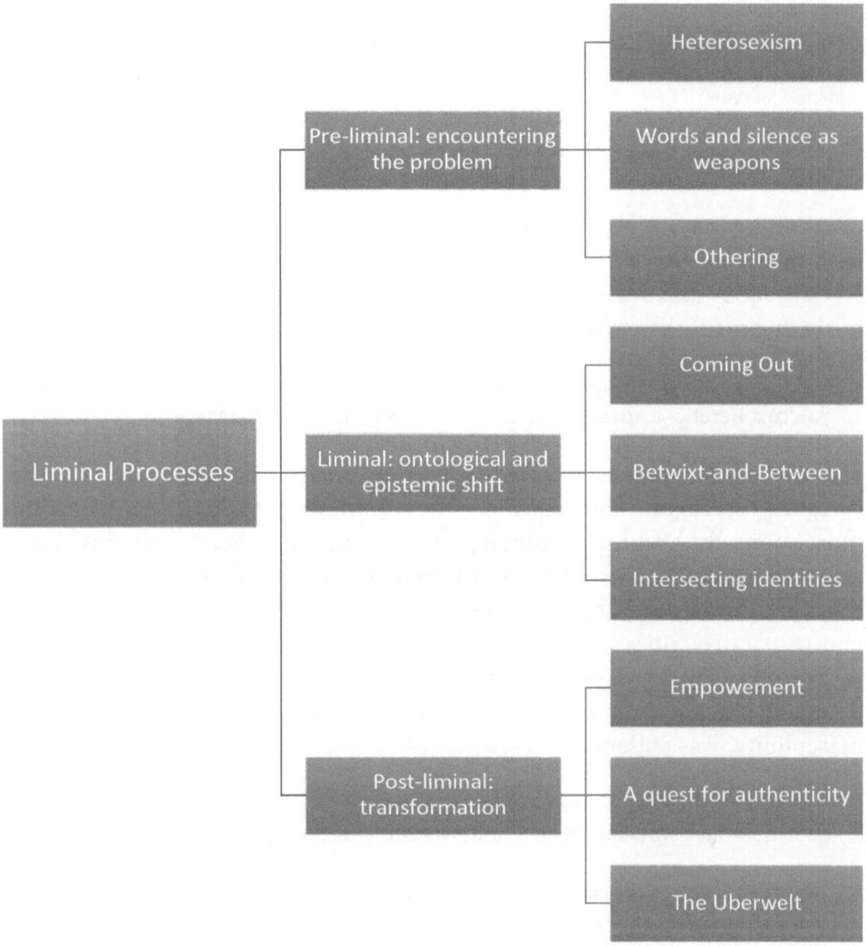

Figure 4. Master theme 2 with sub-themes.

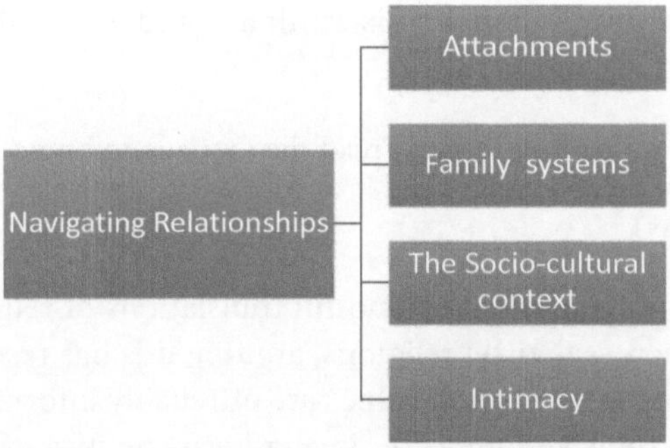

Figure 5. Master theme 3 with sub-themes.

Table 2. Recurrent themes.

Master Theme	*Rose*	*Cate*	*Mark*	*Pam*	*Paul*	*Jay*	Present in over half the sample?
Religious Tribalism	Yes	Yes	Yes	Yes	Yes	Yes	Yes
Liminal Processes	Yes	Yes	Yes	Yes	Yes	Yes	Yes
Navigating Relationships	Yes	Yes	Yes	Yes	Yes	Yes	Yes

religious people are often mystified as to why anyone would choose to align with potentially oppressive institutions.

Orthodoxy and dogmatism were linked in the findings, described humorously by one of the participants:

> Orthodoxy is whichever bully-boy group is stronger than the others. So, if you're a heretic, it means you just weren't strong enough. (Mark)

Schmidt (2011), argues that psychotherapy fits more reasonably into the category of religion and Cormier-Otano and Davies (2012) contend that most counselling and psychotherapy models privilege heterosexuality, both as a social norm and as a sign of psychological health. Davies (2007) claims that practitioners are unlikely to be specifically trained to work with gender and sexual diversities.

The dominant position of men was legitimised by the wider system in the data, and the subordination of women, and any alternative expressions of masculinity, was endemic:

> ... the way that men have silenced women over the years, and it's the male gods that have won-out, men's understanding of their gods. (Mark)

Although gender theory has moved beyond simply examining hegemonic masculinity, with discussion about the multiplicity of masculinities and femininities, the archetypal form of masculinity (i.e. strong, dependable, stoic) remains the most highly valued. Archetypes emerged from religious texts. Participants were expected to have a thorough knowledge of the primary religious text ('The Book'). The misinterpretation of the scripture appeared to give permission to discriminate and reject those who were perceived to be non-compliant.

> ... there's an onus on you to pray, read the Qur'an, and not just read it but interpret the Qur'an and understand it, and act upon it as well ... that's exactly how I learnt. (Jay)

Helminiak (1994) highlights the doubtful translations of religious texts over many years and across theistic religions, arguing this has resulted in generations of people whose beliefs and values are unreliably informed (Helminiak, 1994). There is extensive literature on the hermeneutics of religious texts. Lacoste (2020) points out that despite predating many of the salient texts on this theme, Heidegger (1979) remains a timeless resource for readers seeking to understand the place of God within phenomenology.

Participants' experiences of coming to terms with the apparent conflict between organised religion and homosexual-orientation in the liminal was depicted.

> ... at first it was difficult because I still thought being gay was wrong, you know, 'How am I like this?' because of the tradition I'd been brought up in, because there was no mention of being gay. Well then, 'Did God create me gay?', 'Why has God created me gay?' All those sorts of questions. (Mark)

As an inescapable social ideology, heterosexism was described as implicit and explicit:

> From a young age, all you hear about is that homosexuality is forbidden within Islam, so there is a real taboo to it. You go straight to hell for it.... It's got a real taboo associated with it. (Jay)

Herek (2004) pointed out that conservative religions have been shown across numerous studies to be highly potent predictors of heterosexism. The danger of heterosexism is that it invariably leads to stigmatising and operates through a dual process of silence and attack. Worthington et al. (2002) encourage therapists to reflect on their heterosexual privilege.

Words and silence have consequences in the talking therapies, and these were used as weapons in the religious armoury:

> Unspeakable, yeah. I mean there was always that title 'The love that must never speak its name'. I never talked about it with anybody... so I decided 'well okay, I have to suppress this, and accept the convention route'. (Pam)

Weststrate and McLean (2010) point out that wherever the heterosexual narrative prevails, the gay narrative is silenced. They present a theoretical framework of 'voice and silence' which is based on the dynamics of place and power, emerging as a function of these, both historically and in the present. Lesbian and gay narratives unavoidably subvert and resist dominant conservative narratives, and therefore often silenced.

'Coming out' is an abbreviation of the colloquial phrase 'coming out of the closet' which resulted in a profound ontological and epistemic shift. Participants confronted the shock of almost instantaneously being assigned to a subordinate social category, 'mad, bad, and dangerous to know' (Davies, 2012):

> ... I thought he was a friend. I think if you can turn on a dime like that towards one of the people who worships, who has led worship, has had that much involvement, then there's obviously not much to you. (Paul)

Beckett (2010) recommends 'inviting-in' rather than 'coming-out' since 'inviting-in' provides an alternative perspective to the heteronormative notion of 'the closet'. Moore (2012) highlights that where 'coming out' is a process dependent on a person publicly exiting the closet as an act of resistance or protest, 'inviting-in' is a process that enables self-agency.

As identity dissolved through a growing self-awareness of sexuality, there was initial disorientation but also an awareness of new emergent possibilities:

> I don't know if you know that story of the Velveteen Rabbit? It's a children's story. It's about a toy rabbit that wants to be a real rabbit, and eventually does become a real rabbit. And that's been a constant prayer of mine, 'When am I going to become real?' - when am I going to be able to marry these two things, you know, my gay life, or wanting to be a gay woman, with my faith? (Pam)

McGeorge and Stone-Carlson (2011) stress the need for heterosexual therapists in particular, to become more aware of the influences of everyday heteronormative assumptions, heterosexual privileges, and the impact of heterosexual identities on the therapy process.

Das Nair and Butler (2012) suggest that there is a complex negotiation between aspects of the marginalised self. Jay had to negotiate being a gay, Pakistani, Muslim man within a White, Welsh-speaking school:

> I suppose for me the main difference I felt in school was not from a religious point of view but from a racial point of view ... you had darker skin than everybody else that was there, your culture was different, there were a lot of things you couldn't do that other children could do. (Jay)

Das Nair and Butler (2012) suggest the 'project of intersectionality' will always be incomplete, not only because of the endless possible permutations and combinations of identities and social positions people have, but also because of the changing nature of these identities. In the 'Post-liminal', new aspects of identity formed and empowerment frequently signalled a shift in political perspectives:

> I've done a lot of reading about feminism. Have you come across Camille Panya? She talks a lot about female god religions but also how the male god religions have pretty much suppressed them all. (Mark)

Perkins and Zimmerman (1995) describe empowerment of lesbian and gay people as an ongoing process within communities, in which people are encouraged to actively share resources and increase control over their lives.

Authenticity, the opposite of self-alienation, equated with being true to oneself and being visible:

> There's that element of discovering who you really are again, and the satisfaction you get to know that being gay isn't just about sex but it's about being with somebody, enjoying their company, and being attracted to somebody of the same sex . . . With that, you gradually get more confident to be who you are. (Jay)

Levy and Reeves (2011) note that identity is often understood as unified and authentic, suggesting that in 'finding ourselves' people seek an essential core identity. Taking a flexible, pluralistic perspective, they concur with Clark and Dirkx (2000) who propose that the idea of a unified self does not capture the diversity of personal experiences.

Helminiak (1994) proposed that spirituality may be more about identifying a deeper existential understanding of the self and how that self relates to the world. Participants framed spirituality in different ways including: faith in people, human connectedness, and doing good:

> I do notice there's a huge difference between spirituality and religion, and I feel that I do lots of good. Spirituality is about helping others and that's where my spiritual home is. (Mark)

Lalich and Mclaren (2010) highlight that families with a strong emphasis on traditional family values are less accepting of homosexuality than families who rate low on traditionalism. They argue that a family's religion has a profound effect on parental attitudes towards sexual minority offspring. Figueroa and Tasker (2014) call on therapists to focus on the internalization of negative religious messages transmitted by parents from childhood in order to help young people deal with feelings of self-rejection and self-recrimination.

> Because the more you grow up, the more you're aware, and there are elements of religion within it, but then I suppose there's a lot more of a cultural point of view as well because it comes down to being respected in the community, and it doesn't matter at what cost. (Jay)

Davies (2012) emphasise the power of external oppression regarding sexual orientation, gender, and ethnicity deriving from heteronormative, patriarchal, Eurocentric social influences that lead to internalized oppression. Where same-sex intimacy simply could not be achieved there were negative consequences:

> ... she went back to NZ and I felt completely frustrated. She subsequently divorced her husband, but I lost touch with her, she didn't want to be in touch. I got to the state where I was just at rock-bottom really. (Pam)

When religious leaders and groups reject lesbian and gay people, this negatively affects self-esteem, stifles development, and damages self-acceptance (Barton, 2010).

4.1. Thematic divergences

Although some themes (e.g. shame, judgement, power, silence, and betrayal) are often intertwined, there were subtle thematic divergences noted in these depending on unique religious socio-cultural norms.

5. Conclusion

Socio-political processes that are rooted in religion can reflect in wider social systems, including in the field of psychotherapy. My research highlights the need for heterosexual therapists to be aware of the influences of heteronormative assumptions, heterosexual privileges, and heterosexual identities on both their personal and professional lives.

Although therapists should avoid assuming that lesbian and gay religious clients are necessarily dealing with religious-cultural identity conflict, it is worth reflecting on how to be with clients experiencing such conflicts. Navigating the conflicts that arise at the intersection of sexuality and religion can lead to significantly altered religious beliefs or even in abandoning religious identities entirely. Awareness of a plurality of perspectives regarding sexuality and religious identities is imperative.

Acknowledgements

I express heartfelt thanks to my soulmate José Pizarro, for his love and support. This research project would not have been possible without the guidance of my academic adviser Dr. Sofie Bager-Charleson, to whom I express my thanks and gratitude. Thanks to my supervisor Rusty Livock for her knowledge and wisdom. I express my sincere gratitude to the six extraordinary participants in this research project for engaging so fully with me, and for inviting me in. Also, to all my clients over the years who inspired me to embark upon this work - thank you.

Disclosure statement

No potential conflict of interest was reported by the author.

Funding

The research degree at Metanoia Institute was self-funded.

Data availability statement

The full set of data associated with the paper can be found at: http://mirep.metanoia.ac.uk/id/eprint/212/1/PCMeades%20thesis.pdf

References

Adamczyk, A., & Pitt, C. (2009). Shaping attitudes about homosexuality: The role of religion and cultural context. *Social Science Research*, *38*(2), 338–351. https://doi.org/10.1016/j.ssresearch.2009.01.002

Bachmann, C. L., & Gooch, B. (2018). LGBT in Britain. Health report. *Stonewall (ed.)*. Stonewall/YouGov.

Barton, B. (2010). "Abomination"—Life as a Bible belt gay. *Journal of Homosexuality*, *57*(4), 465–484. https://doi.org/10.1080/00918361003608558

Beckett, S. (2010). Azima ila Hayati: An invitation into my life. Narrative conversations about sexual identity. In Moon, L. (Ed.), *Queer challenges to heteronormativity*. Ashgate.

Bent-Goodley, T. B., & Fowler, D. N. (2006). Spiritual and Religious Abuse. *Journal of Women and Social Work*, *21*, 282–295.

Bowers, R., Minichiello, V., & Plummer, D. (2010). Religious attitudes, homophobia, and professional counselling. *Journal of LGBT Issues in Counselling*, *4*(2), 70–91. https://doi.org/10.1080/15538605.2010.481961

Clark, M. C., & Dirkx, J. M. (2000). Moving beyond a unitary self: A reflective dialogue. In *Handbook of adult and continuing education*. Jossey-Bass.

Clarke, J. M., Brown, J. C., & Hochstein, L. M. (1990). Institutional religion and gay/lesbian oppression. *Marriage & Family Review*, *14*(3–4), 265–284. https://doi.org/10.1300/J002v14n03_13

Cormier-Ontaño, O., & Davies, D. (2012). *Collected papers on GDST 2012/2013*. Pink Therapy International.

Coyle, A., & Rafalin, D. (2000). Jewish gay men's accounts of negotiating cultural, religious, and sexual identity: A qualitative study. *Journal of Psychology & Human Sexuality*, *12*(4), 21–48. https://doi.org/10.1300/J056v12n04_02

Das Nair, R., & Butler, C. (2012). *Intersectionality, sexuality and psychological therapies: Working with lesbian, gay and bisexual diversity*. BPS Blackwell.

Davies, D. (2007, February). Not in front of the students. *Therapy Today*.

Davies, D. (2012). Sexual orientation. In Feltham, C. & Horton, I. (Eds.), *The Sage handbook of counselling and psychotherapy* (3rd ed.). Sage.

Figueroa, V., & Tasker, F. (2014). "I always have the idea of sin in my mind. . . .": Family of origin, religion, and Chilean young gay men. *Journal of GLBT Family Studies*, *10*(3), 269–297. https://doi.org/10.1080/1550428X.2013.834424

Harper, D., & Thompson, A. R. (2012). *Qualitative research methods in mental health and psychotherapy: A guide for students and practitioners*. Wiley-Blackwell.

Heidegger, M. (1979). Heidegger et la question de Dieu. In Lacoste, J. (2020). Heidegger among the Theologians, Journal for Continental Philosophy of Religion, 2(2), 159174. (2), 159174.

Helie, A. (2004). Holy hatred. *Reproductive Health Matters*, *12*(23), 120–124. https://doi.org/10.1016/S0968-8080(04)23114-7

Helminiak, D. (1994). What the Bible really says about homosexuality. In Bowers, R., Minichiello, V., & Plummer, D. (Eds.), *Religious attitudes, homophobia, and professional counselling*. Journal of LGBT Issues in Counselling.

Herek, G. M. (1987). Religious orientation and prejudice: A comparison of racial and sexual attitudes. *Personality & Social Psychology Bulletin, 13*(1), 34–44. https://doi.org/10.1177/0146167287131003

Herek, G. M. (2004). Beyond "homophobia": Thinking about sexual prejudice and stigma in the twenty-first century. *Sexuality Research and Social Policy, 1*(2), 6–24. https://doi.org/10.1525/srsp.2004.1.2.6

King, M., Semlyen, J., Tai, S., Killaspy, H., Osborn, D., Popelyuk, D., & Nazareth, I. (2008). A systematic review of mental disorder, suicide, and deliberate self-harm in lesbian, gay and bisexual people. *BMC Psychiatry, 8*(1), 1–17. https://doi.org/10.1186/1471-244X-8-70

Lacoste, J. (2020). Heidegger among the theologians. *Journal for Continental Philosophy of Religion, 2*(2), 159–174. https://doi.org/10.1163/25889613-00202002

Lalich, J., & Mclaren, K. (2010). Inside and outcast: Multifaceted stigma and redemption in the lives of gay and lesbian Jehovah's witnesses. *Journal of Homosexuality, 57*(10), 1303–1333. https://doi.org/10.1080/00918369.2010.517076

Larkin, M., & Thompson, A. (2012). Interpretative phenomenological analysis. In Thompson, A. & Harper, D. (Eds.), *Qualitative research methods in mental health and psychotherapy: A guide for students and practitioners*. Wiley.

Levy, D. L., & Reeves, R. (2011). Resolving identity conflict: Gay, lesbian, and queer individuals with a Christian upbringing. *Journal of Gay & Lesbian Social Services, 23*(1), 53–68. https://doi.org/10.1080/10538720.2010.530193

McGeorge, C., & Stone-Carlson, T. (2011). Deconstructing heterosexism: Becoming an LGB affirmative heterosexual couples and family therapist. *Journal of Marital and Family Therapy, 37*(1), 14–26. https://doi.org/10.1111/j.1752-0606.2009.00149.x

Melton, J. G. (1991). *The church speaks on: Homosexuality*. Gale Research.

Meyer, I. H., & Dean, L. (1998). Internalised homophobia, intimacy, and sexual behaviour among gay and bisexual men. In Herek, G. M. (Ed.), *Stigma and sexual-orientation: Understanding Prejudice against lesbians, gay men, and bisexuals*. Sage.

Moore, D. (2012). Coming out or inviting in? Part II. *The Feminist Wire* [Online]. Retrieved June 24, 2019, from http://www.thefeministwire.com/2012/07/coming-out-or-inviting-in-part-ii/

Perkins, D. D., & Zimmerman, M. A. (1995). Empowerment theory, research, and application. *American Journal of Community Psychology, 23*(5), 569–579. https://doi.org/10.1007/BF02506982

Reid, K., Flowers, P., & Larkin, M. (2005). Exploring lived experience. *The Psychologist, 18*, 126–136.

Rodriguez, E. M. (2010). At the intersection of church and gay: A review of the psychological research on gay and lesbian Christians. *Journal of Homosexuality, 57* (1), 5–38. https://doi.org/10.1080/00918360903445806

Schmidt, K. (2011). *Not afraid to tell the truth. Exposing apostacy and the conspiracy of silence in the last days*. xlibris.

Shallenberger, D. (1996). Reclaiming the spirit: The journeys of gay men and lesbian women toward integration. *Qualitative sociology, 19*(2), 195–215. https://doi.org/10.1007/BF02393418

Slife, B. D. (2004). Taking practice seriously: Toward a relational ontology. *Journal of Theoretical and Philosophical Psychology, 24*(2), 157–178. https://doi.org/10.1037/h0091239

Smith, J., Flowers, P., & Larkin, M. (2009). *Interpretative phenomenological analysis: Theory, method and research*. Sage.

Super, J. T., & Jacobson, L. (2012). Religious abuse: Implications for counseling lesbian, gay, bisexual, and transgender individuals. *Journal of LGBT Issues in Counseling*, *5*(3–4), 180–196. https://doi.org/10.1080/15538605.2011.632739

Szymanski, D. M., & Chung, B. (2003). Feminist attitudes and coping resources as correlates of lesbian internalised heterosexism. *Feminism & Psychology*, *13*(3), 369–389. https://doi.org/10.1177/0959353503013003008

Unterman, A. (1995). Some orthodox perspectives. In Magonet, J. (Ed.), *Jewish explorations of sexuality*. Berghahn Books.

Weststrate, N., & McLean, K. (2010). The rise and fall of gay: A cultural-historical approach to gay identity development. *Memory (Hove, England)*, *18*(2), 225–240. https://doi.org/10.1080/09658210903153923

Worthington, R. L., Savoy, H. B., Dillon, F. R., & Vernaglia, E. R. (2002). Heterosexual identity development: A multidimensional model of individual and social identity. *Counselling Psychologist*, *30*(4), 496–531. https://doi.org/10.1177/00100002030004002

Yip, A. K. T. (2005). Queering religious texts: An exploration of British non-heterosexual Christians' and Muslims' strategy of constructing sexuality-affirming hermeneutics. *Sociology*, *39*(1), 47–65. https://doi.org/10.1177/0038038505049000

Yip, A. K. T. (2010a). Special feature: Sexuality and religion/spirituality. *Sexualities*, *13*(6), 667–670. https://doi.org/10.1177/1363460710384555

Yip, A. K. T. (2010b). Coming home from the wilderness: An overview of recent scholarship research on LGBTQI religiosity/spirituality in the West. In Browne, K., Munt, S. R., & Yip, A. T. K. (Eds.), *Queer spiritual spaces: Sexuality and sacred spaces*. Ashgate.

Yip, A. K. T. (2014). When religion meets sexuality: Two tales of intersection. In Dickey-Young, P., Shipley, H., & Trothen, T. (Eds.), *Religion and sexuality*. University of British Columbia Press.

Contemporary psychotherapy: Evolution in our modern time

Silva Neves

ABSTRACT
This article is a response to the papers in this special issue. It argues that change and learning is necessary to keep a contemporary psychotherapy practice. However, it asserts that change is also difficult because allowing ourselves to face our 'blind spots' may provoke uncomfortable feelings such as shame. It is therefore important for psychotherapists to be robust in managing the discomfort of learning. With this in mind, the article comments on the papers in this issue, which pay attention to the diversity of our modern populations – including LGBTQ+ people, people of diverse ethnic and racial identities and disabled people. The article argues that by embracing diversity the psychotherapy profession can continue to evolve, enabling it to support diverse communities in the best way possible. It asserts that each of the articles in this special issue invites the reader into a deep self-reflection, helping them to consider all the nuances of difference constructively.

Our modern time

The field of psychotherapy has seen major changes in its conceptualisation and delivery over the last few years. For example, the pandemic has changed how we, and our clients, compare in-person therapy and online therapy. Pre-pandemic, the majority believed that online therapy was not as good and efficient as in-person therapy, making the latter the 'Gold Standard' of therapy. At the beginning of the first UK lockdown, I remember seeing a lot of debates (and arguments) on Twitter about the effectiveness of online therapy. My observation was our colleague's opinions were influenced by two main factors: the modality they were trained in and their level of comfort with technology. Now, almost three years since the pandemic arrived on UK shores, we are continuing to see online therapy flourish and we learned that it is just as powerful and efficient as in-person therapy, yet different. Online therapy is good for clients too. Therapy has become more accessible for disabled people who find difficult it to leave their house or manage the stairs to their therapist's office. Many clients find therapy more convenient to schedule without factoring in the travelling time to the therapist's office. Some therapists can offer cheaper rates when they don't have to pay the high cost of renting a consulting room. Specialist therapists, often concentrated in London and other big cities, are now available for people living in rural areas. Continuous professional development trainings (CPD) were traditionally London-centred before the pandemic, but have now become more accessible and cheaper when delivered online. The adaptation of the psychotherapy profession into the modern world, even if enforced by the pandemic, was outstanding. The landscape of psychotherapy truly changed.

Other major events happened in the last few years. The murder of George Floyd, amongst many other people of diverse ethnic and racial identities, sparked important conversations about institutional racism and previously unchallenged colonial mindsets. People of diverse ethnic and racial identities in our profession started to speak up more, and the rest of us needed to listen. Sadly, I heard many reports of psychotherapy trainees who complained that they were either dismissed or they had to become 'the teacher' in raising awareness working with people who are not white. Disturbingly, some trainees even reported being traumatised by their training.

The same goes for people identifying with diverse gender identities, sexual orientations and relationship styles that do not conform to monogamous heterosexuality. Psychotherapy training organisations tend to offer discussions on case studies that are mostly heterosexual and monogamous. Furthermore, they discuss how to work with these people through a heteronormative lens. The topic of working with LGBTQIA+ people is reserved for a one-day module (if lucky), and serves as a tick-box exercise under the category of 'special populations'. The poor training in gender, sex and relationship diversity (GSRD) is reported as a negative impact on our clients: only 38% of LGBT+ people were satisfied with the mental health services they received from generic support compared to 80% of satisfaction from those accessing LGBT+ specific mental health support (Hubbard, 2021).

Clinicians who are committed to social justice can help the field of psychotherapy to evolve in understanding the greater diversity of humankind. Social justice is challenging the ubiquitous judgmental narratives of our society. If we pay attention to them, they are everywhere. If we don't pay attention to them, therapists can be influenced by those narratives and add to the oppression of our marginalised clients instead of helping them.

It was both heart-warming and exciting to read articles in this journal from authors of various theoretical backgrounds, thoughts and ideas, committed to questioning their attitudes towards diversity and inclusivity. The authors in this journal challenge the traditional psychotherapy status quo by shining the light on our common biases, alerting us of the potential harm of our blind spots, and contribute to the modernisation of our beloved psychotherapy, moving with the times and the diverse populations it serves. Rothschild (2021) writes:

> I have always been of the belief that differing points of view are necessary for the growth and development of any field of study (...) Where there is only agreement, there is stagnation. (2021, p. xvii)

Staying contemporary: The discomfort of ongoing learning

Being, and staying, a contemporary psychotherapist involves a commitment to keep learning and a willingness to let go of some previously accepted theories for new ones when new knowledge becomes more appropriates. Psychotherapy books, especially those with particular ontological positions, are written with the authors' culture, location, their personal and professional positionality, their societal understanding of 'being humans', and the knowledge and limitations of psychology at the time of writing their books. We must understand our theories within the context in which they were written, and allow for what or whom those theories haven't considered. Even science which might be considered 'objective' is constantly evolving with new understanding. Scientists argue and learn from each other. Rothschild (2021) offers more wisdom for us:

> (. . .) science consists of approximations that we use until better ones come along. In no way is this a failure of science (. . .) It is a very normal process of knowledge and professional development. Where it can be a problem is when approximations are taken to be certainty. (2021, pp. xviii-xix)

In other words, being a contemporary psychotherapist is difficult and uncomfortable because we have to walk the very thin line of balancing ourselves between two dimensions: 'I'm a good enough therapist' and 'I have more to learn'. At the same time, being a contemporary psychotherapist is exciting because the discoveries of the human psyche is ongoing and I feel joy in knowing that whatever I write or teach today may be quite different in five years from now.

The commitment to keep learning isn't as easy as it sounds. The four stages of learning, first introduced by Broadwell in 1969 and presented in various iterations since, is a helpful model to identify where we are in our professional development at any given time: (1) unconscious incompetence, (2) conscious incompetence, (3) conscious competence, (4) unconscious competence. These different stages can be hard for a psychotherapist because we know that our competence, or lack of, has a direct impact on our clients' wellbeing. Do we all strive to be at the forth stage? It is a comfortable stage to maintain the illusion that we are at our best and therefore 'always good' for our clients. I argue that to be a good and contemporary psychotherapist, we have to accept the harsh reality that we have to continually move between those four stages. We need to question ourselves and our blind spots. We call them 'blind' because they may be in our unconscious incompetence. Conscious incompetence is very useful to guide us on how to prioritise our CPDs. Conscious competence can help us feel good about ourselves, noticing what theories, methods and interventions work for some clients and not others. Unconscious competence is also useful to celebrate ourselves and our seniority in the profession, while remaining humble by remembering that when we reach that stage, we are still moving through the other stages too. When I deliver training in GSRD, I frequently notice that heterosexual therapists are surprised to learn that 69 countries in the world are inhospitable to LGBTQ+ people (Human Dignity Trust). The privilege of heterosexuality means that they never have to think about their safety if they fancy a holiday in the Middle East, for example, while LGBTQ+ people need to seriously consider the laws of the country they wish to visit. It may seem like a very small detail for heterosexual people, but it is crucially relevant for LGBTQ+ people. The same goes with the seemingly unimportant action of holding hands. An act that heterosexual people never have to think about, but one that may have serious consequences for same-sex couples. When therapists learn something surprising, they stumble on their unconscious incompetence (blind spot) and becoming conscious of it (awareness of their lack of knowledge) may be painful because it can provoke shame (Am I a bad therapist to have had that blind spot?). The Compass of Shame conceptualised by Nathanson (1992) is a good model to remind ourselves in checking our reactions to learning. When we feel shame moving through the stages of learning we might: (1) attack ourselves, (2) attack the trainer, training organisation, or colleagues who have different opinions, (3) withdraw and not learn, (4) dismiss and believe we don't need to learn because we know it all (ie: '*people are people, I treat everybody the same, I don't need a CPD on diversity*').

Indeed, being a contemporary psychotherapist requires uncomfortable, ongoing learning and the management of our shame with self-compassion. I invite the readers of this journal to embrace all their stages of learning and the necessary discomfort that comes with it.

Seeing the invisible

In this special issue, the authors of *Being Seen? The lived experience of psychodynamic practitioners disclosing or not disclosing sight impairment* and *How might psychotherapy improve its service to Disabled people and people with physical impairment* highlight that the field of psychotherapy is ableist, with hardly any literature on disabilities rendering this vast population invisible in our profession.

Sally Parsloe, author of *How might psychotherapy improve its service to Disabled people and people with physical impairment*, writes:

> Psychotherapy stands accused by disability studies of remaining aloof from disability, of failing to offer an alliance, of failing to take account of a significant aspect of human experience, and worse, of actively exacerbating the situation of those people who have bodily impairment

It is important to challenge the psychotherapy profession and its relationship with disability so that we can be more aware of our ableism. Moreover, the paper *Being Seen? The lived experience of psychodynamic practitioners disclosing or not disclosing sight impairment* by Laura Evers explores in much depth the essential – and treacherous – issue of self-disclosure and disability.

The latter points out that therapists with a disability such as sight impairment can be left feeling vulnerable and anxious, and also caught in the confusion of the different opinions on whether their disability should be disclosed to clients or not. The paper analyses the different meanings of being 'client-centred'from both Rogerian and Kleinian perspectives: on the one hand, it can be said that self-disclosure helps the therapeutic alliance;; on the other hand, the anonymity facilitates clients' projections for the purpose of interpretation. So, where do we begin to think about it? Evers positions her discussion, rightly so, on moving away from the permission vs prohibition binary of self-disclosure into a more nuanced terrain of thinking carefully about how the therapist's self-disclosure of their sight impairment might affect the therapeutic process. One of the key aspects of the discussion is to think about how non-disclosure may reinforce the erasure of difference, which can collude with the oppressive societal message of 'normality' and the stigma of impairment. Evers illustrates the problematic erasure of difference with the case of Mary who reported her experience of being treated like everyone else when she needed to be treated differently. This is a common experience amongst minority groups who report that their difference was erased by the therapist's well-intentioned endeavour to 'treat everyone the same'.

Although it can be problematic not to self-disclose, it is also important to seriously consider the impact of self-disclosure, in terms of clients' projections seeing their therapist's vulnerability, perhaps bringing with it feelings around death into the room. We ask our clients engaging in therapy to become vulnerable, but are we doing the therapeutic process a disservice by pretending, or not showing, our own vulnerability? What if 'the work' for some clients is precisely to help them confront their death anxiety through our vulnerability?

Death is often a taboo subject which feels easier to avoid. Evers reflects on the dynamic of 'daring to "be seen" by others' and "Holding clients' need to 'be seen'". The therapist's daring to be seen with their sight impairment (or any other disabilities/vulnerabilities) may be in itself the very holding of their client's need to 'be seen' as they are in the here-and-now (i.e. hearing their anxiety about vulnerability). In other words, clients may find resilience facing their future life adversities through the modelling of the therapist holding their own vulnerability. Being psychologically 'seen' beyond the literal here-and-now may be a profound process.

Evers also describes the unapologetic stance of 'being' disabled and embracing the adaptation to it (through therapy) in the case of Amanda. Her decision to self-disclose became in line with her internal process of self-acceptance. The therapist's relationship to themselves seems to be significant here, which I believe is true for so many of the things we get caught up with in the psychotherapy room whether it be named 'disability' or something else. Amanda's relationship with herself may consciously and unconsciously be of benefit for her clients who struggle with their own self-acceptance. In all cases, Evers asserts that the timing of self-disclosure is of paramount importance, which can be guided through consulting with their supervisors. Because of the lack of psychotherapeutic literature on disability, if the therapist and their supervisor are to discuss the dilemmas of self-disclosure vs non-disclosure, it may require them to find new lenses through which to 'see'.

In *How might psychotherapy improve its service to Disabled people and people with physical impairment, Sally Parsloe* makes an astute point: 'Are not all human bodies restricted in some manner?' giving examples of athlete's bodies performing at a different level than other bodies. Who gets to decide what is 'normal' and what is not? And how do we then decide what is outside of that 'normal' and what is 'dysfunctional'? The best known model of disability is the medical one as it is the dominant narrative in our western societies. It means that people are classified disabled if they are not physically or mentally performing at the level of 'functioning' assessed by the medical standard (Marks, 1997). If, as psychotherapists, we also see our client's disability from that same medical standard, we run the risk of 'not seeing' the person at all. Parsloe writes:

> the individualistic nature of therapy might be seen as an amputation of the client from their world, leading inevitably to a vacuum of understanding. What emerges from that lens is that we can only help the client if we are prepared to get down into the scrum of everyday existence, the disturbing quiddity of the world, rather than remaining in the ivory tower of psychoanalysis or distributing mechanical behaviour alteration therapies.

I couldn't agree more.

The diverse colours of the rainbow

Embracing diversity is not easy because we have to navigate the conflicts that arise from the intersection of different identities. One common conflict is the intersection between the LGBTQ+ identities and religion, brought forward by Peter Meades' paper, *An Exploration of Lesbian and Gay People's Experiences of Religion, and their Implications for Psychotherapy: An Interpretative Phenomenological Analysis (IPA).* Religions, whether they are Christianity, Islam, Judaism, or others, are notoriously strong in the prohibition of 'homosexuality'. At the time of writing this article, as mentioned above, 69 countries criminalise same-sex consensual sexual activities. 11 of those countries impose the death penalty. Those countries are situated in the Middle East and Africa: Afghanistan, Brunei, Iran, Pakistan, Qatar, Saudi Arabia, United Arab Emirates, Yemen, Mauritania, Nigeria and Somalia (Human Dignity Trust). All of these countries use their homophobic religious stance to justify their laws in killing LGBTQ+ people. It is therefore not possible to separate the oppression that LGBTQ+ people face and religion. In the UK, the law protects LGBTQ+ people but violence motivated by religion still goes on.

In the UK, it is illegal to discriminate against what we call 'protected characteristics' which are: age, disability, gender reassignment, marriage and civil partnership, pregnancy and maternity, race, religion or belief, sex and sexual orientation. Therefore, much of the rhetoric then becomes a conflict of 'rights': people who think it is part of their religious rights to hate LGBTQ+

people vs the rights of LGBTQ+ people to live free of fear of discrimination and hate crimes. This tug of war is even more intense when it happens internally: a person identifying as LGBTQ+ and having a religious faith. As a therapist working with such clients, it can be an ethical dilemma in committing to conduct an anti-oppressive practice and being stuck – as much as the client is stuck – in this intersection. The therapist can't collude with either the idea of 'if you're LGBTQ+ you shouldn't be religious' nor 'if you have a faith, it's more important than your sex life, and it's ok to stay in the closet'. It is worth noting here that a study by Grubbs et al. (2019) shows that high religiosity encourages more beliefs that some sexual behaviours are 'wrong' or an illness (the study was done in the context of moral incongruence, where religious people were more likely to call themselves 'porn addict' because of their religious prohibition to masturbation and accessing porn). It is also important to mention that the UK Government reported that many clients who are offered conversion practices to change their sexual orientation to heterosexuality were encouraged by therapists with religious beliefs (UK Government, 2021). So, religion can be seen as a real threat to LGBTQ+ people's wellbeing. On the other hand, the integration of both religious faith and sexual orientations may enhance wellbeing. The big issue is when integration isn't possible.

In my career, I have seen some clients who successfully integrated their religious faith and their sexual orientation mostly through re-interpreting the religious texts or reframing some of their beliefs. But I have also seen those who were desperate to be loved and accepted by their religious communities and never managed to feel that love and acceptance. Not letting go of the hope that their religious communities will somehow change and become loving may increase depression to the level of suicidality. On the other hand, the extreme pain of letting go of that hope, and finding another community that can love and accept them may eventually improve their mental health. Meades cites many relevant references: Yip (2014), Herek (2004), Weststrate and McLean (2010) and Davies (2012) to name a few. I particularly liked the reference to Beckett (2010) who recommends the language of 'inviting-in' rather than 'coming-out' as the latter is part of the heteronormative frame.

The paper *Queer Minds Queer Needs* by Erene Hadjiioannou and Julian-Pascal Saadi expertly demonstrates why there is a crucial need for GSRD-specific training as well as keeping diversity as a core philosophy of practice. The shared history of LGBTQ+ is that the medical psychiatric field pathologised them as a disease. This gave rise to the social justice stance of 'not about us without us': if the psychotherapy profession wants to write or teach about working with LGBTQ+ people, involve the LGBTQ+ communities in doing so. However, the psychotherapy profession needs to take responsibility for their own learning too. Hadjiioannou and Saadi observe:

> Although reflective practice is a core component of psychotherapeutic work, this rarely extends to discussing straightness or cisness. Overlooking these concepts within psychotherapy trainings and health services forces the Queer community to step up once more to educate and create change.

Due to a lack of reflection, I have unfortunately seen too many LGBTQ+ clients being harmed by their previous therapies, and I have read too many articles pathologising their sexual behaviours because of unchecked heteronormativity and a lack of GSRD knowledge. Davies and Neves (2023) have identified core competencies to be a GSRD therapist working effectively with the LGBTQ+ populations : (1) practice a commitment to social justice, (2) demonstrate cultural humility and cultural competence, (3) understanding of the specific adverse effects of oppression, (4) being trauma-informed, (5) gain knowledge of contemporary sexology, (6) integration of core GSRD theories.

With much oppression of homophobia, biphobia and transphobia, both in our clients' childhoods and in their here-and-now, there is plenty of work to be done in supporting our clients' navigating the heteronormative world. But we must also remember that identifying as LGBTQ+ or Queer goes beyond surviving. The magnificent TED Talk from Professor Esben Esther Pirelli Benestad entitled 'Transgifted' teaches us that by standing unapologetically as who we are, and not colluding with 'fitting in', we can embrace our sense of being gifted. Esben Esther Pirelli Benestad spoke in the context of being trans, and we can extend this sentiment to the entire Queer communities: embracing the gift of being Queer and celebrating Queer joy.

The colours of the rainbow have many intersections. In *Towards an Integrative Model of Multicultural Responsiveness*, Daryl Mahon emphasises that cultural competence needs to operate alongside cultural humility in order to be genuinely open to intersectionality. If one doesn't come with the other, it is easy, as Mahon points out, to share a blind spot with the client that keeps being blind because of the assumption of 'knowing each other' when identifying with one similar aspect of intersectionality but forgetting the others. As a therapist identifying as a gay man, I do not assume I understand all gay men's lived experiences, nor do I make an assumption about what it is like to be a client who shares similar experiences to my own. Identifying as LGBTQIA+ also doesn't give me automatic knowledge of all the colours of the rainbow. I, too, have to learn from books dedicated to working with LGBTQIA+ people.

Psychotherapy and diversity

Now that I have discussed the difficulties and the delight of the ongoing learning to embrace diversity in contemporary psychotherapy, I am going to turn my attention to James Sedgwick's paper *Therapy and Diversity – An (un)therapeutic relationship?*

Sedgwick makes a good point that some diversities are in the spotlights: 'race, sex/gender and sexuality receive the most attention' and others may be in the shadow, such as 'people of below average income, intelligence or attractiveness', and making the rather humorous (or sarcastic) comment noting the absence of workshops on 'counselling ugly people'. I absolutely agree that in embracing diversity there should not be a hierarchy of what diversity group is more worthy of discussing over another. However, I would argue that many trans people are economically disadvantaged, and the gay male communities grapple with the intra-community stress of core themes surrounding intelligence, status and attractiveness (Pachankis et al., 2020). The theme of attractiveness is also discussed in psychotherapy specialising in eating disorders because it is an important factor in assessment and treatment. It is also a theme widely discussed when working with women. Some of those parts belong to our diverse intersectionality, and if we are attuned to them, they are not ignored.

As mentioned earlier, reading articles in this journal about many sections of diversity and intersectionality discussed in such depth, from various theoretical viewpoints makes me feel warm. However, Sedgwick's use of the term 'diversity agenda' left me cold. It reminds me how people use the phrase 'the gay agenda' when they refuse to learn and accept this population. The choice of term 'diversity agenda' might be one of the defences against the discomfort in being in-between conscious incompetence and conscious competence of learning. The papers in this journal have argued in their own way that diversity is not an agenda but a core principle that needs to be embedded in our psychotherapeutic knowledge, much like Unconditional Positive Regards and Empathy are.

The very reason why there are more discussions centred on diversity is because the psychotherapy profession has historically been un-diverse, presenting case studies of heterosexual, white, middle-class people, with incorrect assumptions about women (and their sexuality) deeply entrenched in heteronormativity and mononormativity, with unacknowledged misogyny, racism, homophobia, biphobia, transphobia and ableism, as we have seen in this journal's papers.

I appreciate Sedgwick's interests in words and definitions. I share the same interest. I agree that words inform how we think. Yet, while he is trying to make a point about the term 'diversity', he seems to have forgotten to define what he means by 'therapy' as he writes as though all therapies are based on the same assumptions. In fact, different therapies will have vastly different clinical frameworks which seriously influence how the therapists trained in particular modalities view the notion of diversity. For example, traditional psychoanalysis has theories that may encourage problematising people's erotic desire, gender identity and sexual behaviours (including kink and fetishes). On the other hand, modalities such as Gestalt or person-centred therapy have very different points of reference in treating people of diverse backgrounds by preferring not to interpret but allowing clients' process through affirmative exploratory methods or strength-based interventions that are non-pathologising and holistic philosophies. Those types of therapies are very different from one another. Of course, I don't wish to demonise psychoanalysis as I believe we have much to be grateful for its teaching, including its mistakes, and much of its practice has modernised now, but it depends on the individual practitioners who are willing to keep learning.

Sedgwick's argument in 'doing more' vs 'enough' relates to what I explained above in staying in the four phases of our learning, which means that we can both feel 'I'm good enough' and also 'I need to learn more'. One does not need to negate the other. In my view, working effectively with diverse populations is to be able to be culturally humble and to understand that we never know enough; there will be much of clients' intersectionality that we won't know. Being humble means that we can stay alert to our blind spots and take the opportunity to learn more. For example, reading these papers, I learnt more about people with impaired sight, a section of the population I haven't had the opportunity to learn about until now. We don't need to think of ourselves in the binary of 'doing more' vs 'enough'. How about both? While we are 'enough' as therapists we can always do more. We owe this to our clients and to our profession.

I agree with Sedgwick that 'the absence of prejudice is not synonymous with the presence of knowledge'. Indeed, I have met many very qualified and experienced therapists with BACP and UKCP accreditations who have prejudiced thoughts about some sections of the populations: for example: sex workers, people into BDSM or kink, people who have multiple relationships, people who masturbate to pornography. These prejudices are present in spite of the therapist's knowledge. Staying alert to diversity may actually serve as a reminder that there are many unchecked prejudices in our profession – and sometimes, sadly, therapists and their supervisors share the same prejudices.

I'm concerned that Sedgwick believes microaggression is a 'dubious concept'. This is a sad statement because, in my experience, both clinically and personally, microaggression is very much felt by many people who do not fit with the 'normal' imposed by society. Perhaps it is quite 'inconsequential', to use his language, for those who have the privilege of fitting in comfortably. The very fact that people in minority populations are over-represented in mental health services (Stonewall, 2018) is one of the consequences of microaggression.

In the context of LGBTQ+ people, minority stress, defined by Meyer (2003) as (1) experiences of prejudice, (2) expectations of rejection, (3) hiding, (4) Concealing, (5) internalised homophobia, was re-evaluated by Frost et al. (2022) and found that it is still relevant even though there is greater acceptance of LGBTQ+ people, and it is thankfully getting better for younger people. Minority stress is still felt in the LGBTQ+ communities because, unfortunately, homophobia, biphobia and transphobia are still rife. The term 'microaggression' by its very definition is 'micro' and it is easy to miss and/or dismiss it. It is often undetected and unseen by therapists who are not attuned to it. Yet, for those minority populations, microaggression being seen and discussed properly is the very difference that can make therapy successful or not.

Sedgwick seems to imply that what they call the 'diversity agenda' is a conduit for expressing victimhood. I wholeheartedly disagree. It is, in fact, the opposite: we help people become resilient through strength-based strategies. Diversity is not only concerned with LGBTQ+ people, disabled people and people of diverse ethnic and racial identities. It also concerns white heterosexual men. They, too, are vulnerable to a lot of 'male myths' that can cause distress in their lives (also unseen). LGBTQ+ people are vulnerable to the heteronormative world we live in. People of diverse ethnic and racial identities are vulnerable to intrinsic racism. Disabled people are vulnerable to the world constructed with ableism. Women are vulnerable to widespread, everyday misogyny. Different populations, different vulnerabilities.

While Sedgwick may have us believe that the 'diversity agenda' is unfounded and taking over our profession, it is worth re-balancing the paper with some reality. It is indeed the case that there is a growing number of books, papers and trainings that focus on working with diversity and minority populations like gender, sexuality, race, neurodiversity and disability but, still, it is a small number compared to the majority of books and trainings that are embedded in heteronormative, mononormative, cisgenderist, ableist and white theories. Unfortunately, those theories do not always work, and, in fact, can oppress those who have different identities and cultures.

The language of psychology: Serving clients or psychotherapists?

In *Deconstructing Humanitarian Compassion: Ψ as Method, Artemis Christinaki* discusses the notion of an oppressive practice conceptualised as the 'emotional hospitality'. In the context of refugees and the Christian humanitarian movement,*Christinaki* makes an astute point that refugees have to learn to speak the language of psychology which is then perceived as more civilised. Therapy becomes the new version of confession which must happen for the refugee to be accepted:

> Taking into consideration that refugees do not articulate their suffering in a psychological discourse, as it is a very westernised project of comfort, they are trained to speak in the Other's discourse. Learning to speak a new language, the language of psychology within the neutral zone of humanitarian compassion, an 'emotional hospitality' opens to the psyche, to situate the self efficiently in the new terrain

Christinaki also states:

> While truth is guaranteed in the speaking subject and in the evidence that brings along in the discourse of his statement, the agency of domination does not lie in the one who confess but in the partner who listens. Having set the scene under which the hospitality will take place, the discourse of truth takes effect

This reminded me how some therapists (the one who listens) can dominate their clients by offering interpretations that may be harmful to them. In a different context from the one this paper is based on, I remember a client who identified as a transman telling me that their previous therapist asserted that their desire to transition into a man was because of their 'internalised misogyny' and would do better by learning to be an 'assertive woman'. This led the client not to pursue gender-affirming therapy for over ten years, during which time their distress increased to the point of attempting suicide. When therapists are not aware of their position of power and dominance and treat their marginalised clients as needing to educate them to be 'more civilised' (or to become more like the therapist), harm can occur. Sadly, the anecdote of my transman identified client is not an isolated case. Sex workers are often automatically labelled as 'victims' or pathologised as mentally ill for choosing their profession. People who have more sex than their therapists are labelled 'sex addicts', and so on.

Christinaki's point about psychologising clients and educating them to speak our language makes me reflect on the language we use between us, particularly the one that therapists have with their supervisor. When a therapist tells their supervisor that they struggle with a client because they're not 'psychologically-minded' I am now wondering if the expectation of the therapist (and the supervisor) may be that the client has to learn the language of the therapist before the therapist can actually listen.

This thought-provoking paper makes me think about the other 'spaces' where a therapeutic process can occur that may not be in the westernised ideas of the consulting room. In some cultures, people may psychologically process their pain and angst in the kitchen, making and sharing food together. How about the cultures who drum and dance as their therapeutic process? Drumming may not be as far off as the psychological package of the method we call EMDR (Eye Movement Desensitisation Reprocessing) because drumming involves bilateral movements. Dancing may be processing through body movements, which can be the non-clinical version of recognised western body psychotherapies such as somatic experiencing. We keep all psychological techniques, interventions and practices within the four walls of the consulting room (some of us may venture into 'walking therapy') but we tend to look down on drumming, dancing and being together in the kitchen as validated forms of therapeutic engagements. At best, we might call these activities 'hobbies' or 'self-care'. Self-care is another westernised packaging of the conceptualisation of the functioning of our psyche. Somehow, 'self-care' is presented as support for the 'real' therapeutic process (which must happen in the consulting room) rather than as a therapeutic process as and of itself.

The language we use is so important and powerful. Returning to the topic of refugee clients, Nicole Chew-Helbig offers us a beautifully written case study in her paper,*A Psychotherapist's Lived Experience In-Session with an Asylum Seeker and Translator: An Autoethnographic Case Study*. Despite so much anxiety in the triangle of the client, therapist and translator, there was a meeting of mind, using creativity and human connection beyond the traditional protocols of psychotherapy. I couldn't agree more with her thoughts:

> The mono-personal approach to diagnosis, a dominant paradigm of psychiatry and the DSM, focuses the treatment of symptoms experienced by the individual, while the bi-personal approach of relational modalities of psychotherapy affirms therapeutic change to arise through the therapeutic alliance

With this in mind, allow me to loop back to the papers mentioned earlier. In *Being Seen? The lived experience of psychodynamic practitioners disclosing or not disclosing sight impairment*, Evers rightly debates and questions how the therapist may adapt their practice and challenge the traditional status quo of non-disclosure that is typical with psychodynamic/psychoanalysis theories, while Parsloe, author of *How might psychotherapy improve its service to Disabled people and people with physical impairment*, encourages us to adopt 'the will to self-critique'. Indeed, it is only with that will and our awareness of our multiple layers of conscious and unconscious competence that we can continue to check our fluid process of learning. Embracing diversity in our practice helps avoid unintentional harm to *all* our clients and it can also provide therapists a space to help each other reflect on how we can change and adapt to the evolving world and the needs of diverse populations.

Daryl Mahon, author of *Towards an Integrative Model of Multicultural Responsiveness*, makes an interesting and exciting statement:

> The multicultural competency (MCC) movement can be considered the fourth force in psychotherapy, following on from the psychodynamic, behavioural and humanistic traditions

The author emphasises the importance of intersectionality as a theoretical philosophy. He goes on to say:

> Take two individuals sharing the same race, the intersect of sexuality, socio-economic status or gender can provide for very different experiences of racial identity

Mahon advocates for the idea of pluralism:

> clients may have different culturally specific ideas of how treatment should work, and what type of approaches and methods will be helpful

This is when it is important to challenge and adapt our westernised practice to be more attuned to clients' needs. For example, for an Asian client, the 'self' may mean a collective self not an individualistic one. For some, putting their parents or their position in the family as a priority and above their individual self could be a place of wellbeing, but seen as problematic for the western therapist. Even within Europe, our western theories may not match the healing processes that some cultures adopt. I'm in agreement with Mahon when he writes:

> the Western world's diagnostic system of pathologizing, is certainly not consistent with all cultures, nor is the individualistic approach to therapy

For example, grieving the loss of a loved one is done differently in Greece, Spain, France and Britain. Some cultures may embrace the visibility of mourning as much as crying and wailing while other cultures are less comfortable with it. The period of 'accepted' mourning also differs from one country to the next and may not match with the clinical definition of 'prolonged' or 'complicated' grief 'disorder' according to the ICD-11 (WHO, 2019) and DSM-5 (2013). Yet, there are some universal 'truths' too, for example, that the intensity of grief depends on the quality of the relationship with the dead person.

Concluding thoughts

Here, I would like to mention Tony McSherry's article, *Diversity and aggression: a reflection on sensual meanings and an ameliorative law after Freud and Lacan*, whose concluding thoughts, as uncomfortable as it may be, is a pertinent one to consider:

> Ask yourself what you will do when you have achieved diversity: Will you enclose it? Will only certain others be allowed in to the enclosure? People who think like you? If we are really honest the answer to that question could well be a 'yes'.

As we strive for diversity, we also need to think about boundaries based on different aspects that may not always fit together: clinical evidence, cultural competence, cultural humility, social justice, the awareness of oppression, and so on. We need to think about what we will include and exclude in our practice. The author's invitation in the 'enclosure' of diversity made me think about my own. I exclude some countries' cultural and religious discourse that 'homosexuality' is a disease and refuse to offer conversion practices. I reject the thinking that female genital mutilation is a cultural practice (also, it is illegal in the UK). I will not include clinicians who think opposingly on t these topics as part of my professional network and 'enclosure'. However, I welcome the inclusion of clinicians disagreeing with me on other matters, and I embrace interesting conversations on new thoughts and discoveries about our human mind. I invite the readers of this journal to keep thinking and keep learning about diversity, embracing the evolution of psychotherapy in our modern time. When we keep learning, we keep refining for ourselves and our clients what it means to be alive.

Disclosure statement

No potential conflict of interest was reported by the author.

References

Beckett, S. (2010). Azima ila hayati: An invitation into my life. Narrative conversations about sexual identity. In L. Moon (Ed.), *Queer challenges to heteronormativity*. Ashgate.

Broadwell, M. M. (1969). Teaching for learning. *The Gospel Guardian*, *20*(41), 1.3a.

Davies, D. (2012). Sexual orientation. In C. Feltham & I. Horton (Eds.), *The Sage handbook of counselling and psychotherapy* (3rd ed.). Sage.

Davies, D., & Neves, S. (2023). Gender, sex and relationship diversity therapy. In T. Hanley & L. Winter (Eds.), *The SAGE handbook of counselling and psychotherapy* (5th ed.). Sage

DSM-5. (2013). *Diagnostic and statistical manual of mental disorders* (5th ed.). American Psychiatric Association. American Psychiatric Publishing.

Esben Esther Pirelli Benestad TED Talk: Transgifted. https://youtu.be/H6blufLgo_U

Frost, D. M., Fingerhut, A. W., & Meyer, I. H. (2022). Social change and relationship quality among sexual minority individuals: Does minority stress still matter? *Journal of Marriage and Family, 84*(3), 920–933. https://doi.org/10.1111/jomf.12827

Grubbs, J. B., Kraus, S. W., & Perry, S. L. (2019). Self-reported addiction to pornography in a nationally representative sample: The roles of use habits, religiousness, and moral incongruence. *Journal of Behavioral Addictions, 8*(1), 88–93. https://doi.org/10.1556/2006.7.2018.134

Herek, G. M. (2004). Beyond "homophobia": Thinking about sexual prejudice and stigma in the twenty-first century. *Sexuality Research and Social Policy, 1*, 6–24. https://doi.org/10.1525/srsp.2004.1.2.6

Hubbard, L. (2021). *The hate crime report 2021: Supporting LGBT+ victims of hate crime.* Galop.

Human Dignity Trust. https://www.humandignitytrust.org

Marks, D., (1997). Models of disability. *Disability and Rehabilitation, 19*(3), 85–91. https://doi.org/10.3109/09638289709166831

Meyer, I. H. (2003, September). Prejudice, social stress, and mental health in lesbian, gay, and bisexual populations: Conceptual issues and research evidence. *Psychological Bulletin, 129*(5), 674–697. https://doi.org/10.1037/0033-2909.129.5.674. PMID: 12956539; PMCID: PMC2072932.

Nathanson, D. L. (1992). *Shame and pride: Affect, sex, and the birth of the self.* W.W. Norton & Company.

Pachankis, J. E., Clark, K. A., Burton, C. L., Hughto, J. M. W., Bränström, R., & Keene, D. E. (2020). Sex, status, competition, and exclusion: Intraminority stress from within the gay community and gay and bisexual men's mental health. *Journal of Personality and Social Psychology, 119*(3), 713–740. https://doi.org/10.1037/pspp0000282

Rothschild, B. (2021). *Revolutionizing trauma treatment. Stabilization, safety, & nervous system balance.* W.W. Norton & Company, Inc.

Stonewall. (2018). *LGBT in Britain.* Health Report. https://www.stonewall.org.uk/system/files/lgbt_in_britain_health.pdf

UK Government. (2021). *Conversion therapy: An evidence assessment and qualitative study.* https://www.gov.uk/government/publications/conversion-therapy-an-evidence-assessment-and-qualitative-study/conversion-therapy-an-evidence-assessment-and-qualitative-study#what-forms-does-conversion-therapy-take-1

Weststrate, N., & McLean, K. (2010). The rise and fall of gay: A cultural-historical approach to gay identity development. *Memory, 18*(2), 225–40.

World Health Organization. (2019). *International statistical classification of diseases and re-lated health problems* (11th ed.). https://icd.who.int/

Yip, A. K. T. (2014). When religion meets sexuality: Two tales of intersection. In P. Dickey- Young, H. Shipley, & T. Trothen (Eds.), *Religion and sexuality.* University of British Columbia Press.

Diversity in counselling & psychotherapy

Gillian Proctor

ABSTRACT
This paper is a commentary on the articles in this special issue on diversity and inclusion. The concepts of diversity and inclusion are critiqued, and a critical diversity approach is promoted. The difficulties and strengths for the profession of counselling and psychotherapy adopting this approach are explored. Ableism is raised as an issue with a plea for ongoing deconstruction of language and attention to inequalities both within and without the profession.

Introduction

In this commentary prompted by engaging with the papers in this special issue, I critique the way that diversity and inclusion concepts can be used and recommend a critical diversity approach. I explore some difficulties for the profession of Counselling & Psychotherapy (C&P) in adopting a critical diversity agenda and suggest that we are nevertheless well-prepared for this work, in coherence with our tradition of self and intersubjective awareness. I raise the issue of ableism as a particular example of the necessity for a constant deconstruction of language and attitudes if we are to truly challenge inequalities within and beyond the profession. I weave the papers from this special issue throughout, wherever they are relevant.

Diversity: Celebrating difference or challenging inequalities?

I argue in Proctor (2011, p. 231) that 'The rhetoric of diversity and difference depoliticize the inequalities in society. Linguistic equality cannot change material reality. Embracing the diversity rhetoric is in danger of obscuring inequalities and thus further perpetuating the structures of power in society'.

It is now even clearer to me how the rhetoric of diversity has become a tick-box exercise for many organisations, or an add-on for when we have extra time or energy, often too focused on 'celebrating' or even exoticizing difference (e.g. promoting annual calendar reminders of particular groups such as Pride), rather than the responsibility for constant hard work challenging -isms, prejudice and discrimination whenever we encounter it; in institutions, amongst those around us and in society at large.

I am referring to the difference between the standard organisational 'equality and inclusion' approach with the goal of treating everyone equally (or even equitably); as opposed to a critical focus on each of our own internalisations of societal dualisms which inevitably result in inequalities and prejudices. If the focus is the latter (a critical diversity approach), we are required to constantly be troubling ourselves and others, questioning our own attitudes, assumptions and perceptions of others and noticing what our language and behaviour are revealing of our internal worlds. It requires a commitment to being, for example, anti-racist rather than convincing ourselves and others that we are not racist. Becoming anti-racist starts from the opposite position – knowing we have internalised the racist society we are in and actively working to counteract this impact. Layla Saad (2020) clarifies that challenging racism does not involve trying not to be racist, but instead, to be anti-racist, we must be prepared to lose our privileges – and this means the privilege of not having to challenge whenever others are oppressed.

Critical diversity involves being anti-sexist, anti-heterosexist, anti-ableist and anti-classist among others. It means committing to a critical stance against many of the pillars which prop up mainstream society, including being critical of the factors which supposedly comprise good mental health (such as marriage, monogamy, working in a high-status job, being rational, having an emotionally close family, having no impairments etc). It means creating communities of therapists, organisations and training programmes that question implicit assumptions in our society; including biases towards what attributes make a good therapist. It doesn't stop with the internal work of challenging our own perceptions; but being critical in this way helps us to notice the prejudices of others both individually and organisationally, which result in material inequalities such as access to money, housing, employment, and healthcare.

In the paper *Therapy and Diversity – An (un)therapeutic relationship?*, James Sedgwick questions how C&P adopts the diversity agenda, calling for more attention to material inequalities rather than psychological and relational hurt. However, rather disappointingly, the author then focuses his attention on the critical diversity agenda, arguing that other groups deserve equal attention to the oft-focused-on dynamics of racism and heterosexism. His point would be worth considering if he told us how C&P rarely considers class (see Kearney, 2018) and how we could better meet the needs of the 'people of below average income, intelligence or attractiveness' and their associated disadvantages. However, instead he seems to blame the profession for taking on the anti-racist and queer focus of the diversity agenda. Divisive tactics within groups at the sharp end of inequalities serve no one except those in power who are happy to watch those suffering fight amongst themselves. He would do well instead to be grateful to the 'venerable civil rights movements' whom he mentions and apply the scholarship and activism developed from such movements to other equally deserving groups. We need whatever strategies we have in our critical deconstructing mission, and critical race theory and queer theory are essential areas of scholarship that have forged ahead in challenging dominant discourses in a myriad of ways. It serves no one to wait until all under-represented groups have been acknowledged before creating new ways of exploring the territory.

Inclusion? In dominant society?

Why aim to be included in something which warrants critique? Assimilation is the equivalent of inclusion. It challenges nothing and instead tries to argue for a place at the table by following the dominant discourses. Inclusion fails to change the rules of inequality and structure of society; instead, it just widens the scope of those who have protection. Wouldn't it be better to try to change the rules of the game?

Yet of course all humans need to be included in basic human rights to feel part of humanity. Nevertheless, asking to be included demeans those asking, and leaves power in the hands of the dominant majority. Those in power can then allow or refuse inclusion, with permission often being granted on the condition that they make up for clear identity deficiencies (such as assimilation by changing language and customs). Instead, how can we start from the point of knowing our rights to exist for ourselves and asserting our ways of doing that, however differently? Sethi (2021) demonstrates this powerfully in her discussion on reclaiming her country as hers, against racism. She derives the roots of reclamation from the Latin, referring to a cry of 'no', and begins from the position not of asking to be included but of saying 'I belong here'.

Difficulties for C&P in adopting a critical diversity agenda

I have identified three particular difficulties that C&P must address to take on a truly activist stance in relation to inequalities. These are (1) the ignoring of material realities, (2) the focus on empathic understanding which does not require similar experiences and (3) the historical and current involvement of the profession in the dominant societal agenda to perpetuate inequalities.

Taking material realities seriously

C&P focus on individual and relational reasons for distress. Inequalities result in material deprivation and fear of violence, not just psychological harm. To take a critical diversity approach involves taking the bodily and material inequalities seriously, rather than reducing everything to relational or individual psychology, a point made clearly by James Sedgwick and in Proctor (2006).

Acknowledging the benefits of understanding from experience

How can we respond to clients' wishes to be understood by someone who shares some of their experiences rather than empathic understanding from someone in a very different position? Again, Sedgwick draws attention to the idea that therapist-matching can be useful for clients and can only be possible in teams where therapists are specifically recruited to match their client groups. The danger is that we become defensive about not sharing experiences and argue that this isn't necessary for empathy, rather than acknowledging that different understandings arise from the sharing of experiences. Counselling often focuses on the dangers of understanding from one's own experience (such as identification and assuming similarity. The logic follows that by not conflating one's experience with the client's experience, the counsellor is uniquely placed to empathically understand all clients. However, we also need to acknowledge the different benefits from sharing experiences.

Goffman (1986) refers to 'the own' and 'the wise', as two groups that can be helpful to address stigma. The 'own' are those who share a stigma and the wise are allies, who try to understand the experiences of the stigmatised group from the outside. C&P can work hard to be the 'wise' for stigmatised groups, but this does not need to be at the expense of validating the different contributions of the 'own'.

Towards an Integrative Model of Multicultural Responsiveness by Daryl Mahon addresses many of the critiques of a cultural competency framework, especially the focus on knowledge of diverse cultures. The model includes client preference accommodation (often therapist matching). Mahon reminds us that however hard we try to understand the other, they will always 'overflow' our understanding (Levinas) and this requires an ongoing attitude of humility and not knowing. The model also includes (based on reviews of research) the importance of actively seeking feedback from clients to check how our offerings are received whilst trying to address ruptures before the client drops out.

C&P and psychology reinforcing inequalities

Therapy theories often reinforce inequalities rather than challenge them. These theories are associated with all the norms of societies at the time they originated. Women, black people and disabled people were clear second-class citizens and these ideas are implicit in many theories. Even for those therapy theories such as client-centred therapy (Rogers, 1959), which didn't prioritise any kind of humans over others, autonomy is prioritised over collectivity in accordance with white western values. I argue in Proctor (2006) that therapy is often help for those who least need it and as such is in danger of perpetuating inequalities. As the current mental health crisis deepens and services such as IAPT (Improving Access to Psychological Therapy, see Proctor & Hayes, 2017; Proctor et al., 2020) process clients in superficially numerical ways, only those with money can pay for truly relational therapy. If they can't pay for it, they are likely to come into contact with under-resourced and overwhelmed mental health services.

Psychology arose from a societal context for the purposes of assessing and pathologizing people; a tool to bolster the norms of society (see Newnes, 2014; Rose, 1985). From this academic tradition, the professions of counselling and psychotherapy arose. Similarly, C&P can serve a useful purpose for society to individualise problems by encouraging self-regulation through 'confession'. This reinforces relations of power in society (in a Foucauldian sense, see Proctor, 2017). Whereas most of us enter the profession believing our 'help' to be benign, the implications of this 'help' for society are crucial to examine.

Artemis Christinaki in *Deconstructing Humanitarian Compassion: Psychology as Method* takes up this theme and usefully reminds us of another specific and broader context within which the profession of C&P is situated – that of humanitarian aid. Christinaki argues that the notion of compassion in humanitarian aid arose from the history of colonialism and evangelical Christianity. Today, it can be said that the psycho-social role of supporting refugees similarly encourages a 'confession' (in Foucauldian terms), thus enforcing the identity of the refugee as 'other'. Christinaki argues that the 'hospitality' offered by such humanitarian aid models is anything but hospitable in the Derridean sense, and is in fact 'inhospitable' by clearly inscribing the power relations of host and guest within a country. This article made clear to me my discontent with the concept of 'compassion' and the power relations implicit within it. I understood Christinaki to be suggesting rather than approaching the other from a 'helping' perspective. We need to 'reconstitute the borderland of our selves with the Other and let a dialectic of ... struggle begin. It may be there that dignity lies, while guests and hosts identities start to become loose and elusive'. This resonates with my critique of the inclusion agenda above.

Queer Minds Queer Needs by Erene Hadjiioannous and Julian-Pascal Saadi reminds us how non-conformity in gender, sexuality and relationships has not just been disapproved of socially but taken on by the medical and psychotherapy fields as pathological, including most notably the practice of conversion therapy. Thus, it is incumbent on C&Ps to show our position as queer-affirming, rather than assuming that not taking up a position will be perceived as acceptance. They emphasise the need for therapists to think fluidly not binarily, and for us all to question our own identities with respect to gender and sexuality, especially when our fitting in with dominant categories has overlooked the need to question ourselves.

Peter Meades' *An Exploration of Lesbian and Gay People's Experiences of Religion, and their Implications for Psychotherapy: An Interpretative Phenomenological Analysis (IPA)* reminds us of the difficulties for stigmatised groups to exist within institutions that represent dominant conservative views in society – in this case, religions. The themes looked promising but the discussion and implications of these themes were disappointing. The conclusion is for therapists to be aware that there can be conflict between the heterosexism of conservative religions and living a queer life. I was hoping to hear a more nuanced view of how people negotiate these intersectionalities or subvert the dominant views of religions. It points to the difficulties of fighting for inclusion in systems that are antithetical to the values and existence of such groups.

How C&P could be prepared for the critical diversity agenda

The focus in C&P of ongoing commitment to self and intersubjective awareness can be a big strength in our ability to adopt a critical diversity agenda. One of the difficulties with the equality and diversity agenda in organisations is the focus on training which tries to teach employees to not be biased.Organisations try to ensure that recruitment processes treat all applicants equally rather than discriminating on the basis of characteristics, particularly those protected under the Equality Act (2010). However, such training is rarely more than superficial (see Prasad & Mills, 1997) and can result in employees who know well what we 'should' say to fulfil the organisational agenda of not being discriminatory, with deeply held biases and prejudices remaining firmly intact nevertheless. To truly challenge these societal beliefs that we have all internalised without choice involves deep and ongoing conscious work. It requires a commitment to noticing how our language gives away our often unconscious biases. It requires that we consider the impact of our biases on particular identities. And it involves challenging the false justifications on which these inequalities are based. This work should fit nicely with the commitment expected of C&Ps to ongoing self and intersubjective awareness, with the necessary addition of understanding our intersubjectivity in a societal context. This requires us to take individual responsibility for ongoing awareness, rather than expecting training providers to do it all for us. However, it does still require training providers to emphasise the professional responsibility to self-examine, rather than focusing purely on ideas of competency.

However, McSherry is not so optimistic about this. He argues in his paper, *Diversity and aggression: a reflection on sensual meanings and an ameliorative law after Freud and Lacan*, that Freud's understanding of how we turn away from parts of ourselves leads to an inevitable turning away from others. He argues that the aggression of exclusion is necessary for society (from Freud) and to be honest about this, at the same time implying the necessary personal work to allow more of oneself to acceptance and therefore more of others. His conclusion I find depressing that inclusion will always exclude those most different from ourselves, starting and finishing with fear and defence. I prefer to find the room for exploration of alterity and creativity when there is enough safety. I would also argue against Freud's ideas of what needs to be repressed for the sake of society and suggest that society is in a different position now and that it is repression and exclusion that is the danger.

Ableism

I am frequently surprised by how often ableist language is used within the C&P profession without awareness, and how infrequently it is challenged. Dominant ways of perceiving (seeing and hearing) are conflated with awareness (in phrases such as being 'blind' or 'deaf' to issues);physical presence or voice are conflated with being acknowledged or counted ('to make your voice heard', 'standing up for something') and 'madness' is used routinely to imply irrationality.

Agosto et al. (2019) draw attention to this issue in critical racism, reminding us how vigilant we need to be to not promote the legitimacy of one group at the expense of another. This has been a regular strategy within identity politics and activism, resulting in the acceptance of some members of marginalised groups on the condition that they behave in ways acceptable to dominant values. Thus, married gay people have achieved an acceptance of their relationships and status in society not shared by non-married queer people, and people who experience racism experience more acceptance when they speak with a Received Pronunciation accent (perceived to be 'standard English') as opposed to any culturally specific accent.

Agosto et al. (2019, 38) instead call for 'crippin and queering the curriculum' (see McRuer, 2006), 'requiring one to read differently and reject so-called "best practices" that amount to heteronormative, ableist, individualistic, neoliberal conditions for inclusion. Such practices and conditions can be resisted using crip arts of failure, namely fortunate failure, which is to fail at being assimilated under the guise of inclusion'. This is the approach not of assimilation but of deconstruction and opening a space for thinking differently. People try and prove their 'sanity' and their body as worthy. This proving by trying to fit in with 'normality' both oppresses and marginalises those who fail or refuse, and confers only a conditional acceptance on those who comply. How can we argue for equal worthiness without trying to show similarities to those who are automatically assumed worthy? How do we hold onto our humanity, or being purely alive (to take a less androcentric view), as being enough to prove our right to an existence that accords respect?

This critique is of particular relevance to the paper on therapist self-disclosure by sight-impaired therapists, *Being Seen? The lived experience of psychodynamic practitioners disclosing or not disclosing sight impairment*. The author, Laura Evers, draws our attention to how tenacious disabled therapists need to be in monitoring their own and their client's responses to their impairment, acknowledging their client's fears of vulnerability, death and not being seen, at the same time as monitoring their own potential disavowal of impairment. She emphasises the importance of seeing oneself and others in all our complexity, which she terms as 'bi-abled', having unable and able parts. This article also reminds us of the battle for legitimacy that so many minoritised therapists must fight within training institutions and organisations, which gets in the way of how we might offer the best therapy for our clients. However, the author fails to critique the theoretical focus within C&P theory of being seen, which uses a 'deficit-laden construct ... infer[ring] normative abilities'; instead she could offer alternatives such as being noticed, acknowledged, or understood. There seems to be a missed opportunity in accepting clients' need to be seen rather than a reframing of what this means from a non-normative perceptual stance.

In her article *How might psychotherapy improve its service to Disabled people and people with physical impairment*, Sally Parsloe points to the work we have to do as therapists to deconstruct our theories and practices with respect to ableism and consider seriously our own blocks to approaching the other with respect and awe, particularly when we are privileged and our client is marginalised in some way. The author calls for a shake-up of our theories and a focus on not just internal psychological issues but an interest in our clients as unique others and as bodies in a particular world. This is consonant with the concept of cultural humility and a not-knowing stance (see Proctor, Cahill, et al., 2021).

Engaging people in otherness

The article with which I most engaged was the autoethnography of therapy with an asylum seeker and translator. The author, Nicole Chew-Helbig creates a beautiful narrative that does not seek to control nor explain but to simply be present with another. Her writing encourages people to come 'face-to-face' with the Other in a Levinasian sense, whereby one encounters alterity with curiosity and welcome. (see Proctor, Cahill, et al., 2021).

This led me to consider the use of accusational tactics in dealing with privilege, and the hardening of divisions which they so often cause; whereas a personal story shared with emotion and humility can invite others to engage in a less threatening way. I was reminded of my work in bringing anti-racism to the counselling curriculum. The task was to go beyond people's defences towards authentic encounters, and to notice the empathic challenges and subtle interplays which this entails. (see Proctor, Smith, et al., 2021). However, it does require the tricky negotiation of how not to exploit people in the telling of their stories for the benefit of others (see Denyer et al., 2022).

Conclusion

In order to become a critical approach, diversity and inclusion work needs to move away from 'celebrating differences'. Challenging binaries, inequalities and fixed identities is essential to the development of the counselling and psychotherapy profession. At the same time C&Ps need to acknowledge and welcome the other from a position of shared humanity and seek to learn from alterity (see Proctor, 2019). A critical diversity approach is an approach of not-knowing, adopting a curious, respectful stance for all clients, along with a commitment to ongoing awareness of material inequalities, structural oppressions and embodied existences. Furthermore, in our profession and our training institutes, we need to represent this critical stance as anti-racist; queering, cripping and deconstructing the normative dominant discourses which we have individually and professionally internalised. In doing this ongoing reflective and activist work, we can come closer to creating a place for belonging in diverse ways, reclaiming our lands, our society and the terrain of psychotherapy for all.

Disclosure statement

No potential conflict of interest was reported by the author.

References

Agosto, V., White, A., & Valcarlos, M. M. (2019). Deficit-Laden use of constructs in anti-oppressive curriculum. *Journal of Curriculum Theorizing, 34*(1), 36–49.

Denyer, T., Wade, K., Whitney, M., Charura, D., & Proctor, G. (2022). 'Listen with love': Exploring anti-racism dialogue in psychotherapy and counselling training.

Psychotherapy & Politics International, 20(1 & 2). https://doi.org/10.24135/ppi.v20i1and2.06

Goffman, E. (1986). *Stigma: Notes on the management of a spoiled identity*. New York, NY: Simon & Schuster (Original work published 1963).

Kearney, A. (2018). *Counselling, class and politics: Undeclared influences in therapy* (G. Proctor, Ed.; 2nd ed.). PCCS Books.

McRuer, R. (2006). *Crip theory: Cultural signs of queerness and disability*. NYU press.

Newnes, C. (2014). *Clinical psychology: A critical examination*. PCCS Books.

Prasad, P., & Mills, A. (1997). From showcase to shadow: Understanding the Dilemmas of managing workplace diversity. In P. Prasad, A. Mills, M. Elmes, & A. Prasad (Eds.), *Managing the organizational melting pot: Dilemmas of workplace diversity* (pp. 3–28). Sage.

Proctor, G. (2006). Therapy: Opium for the masses or help for those who least need it? In G. Proctor, M. Cooper, P. Sanders, & B. Malcolm (Eds.), *Politicising the person-centred approach: An agenda for social change* (pp. 66–79). PCCS Books.

Proctor, G. (2011). Diversity: The depoliticization of inequalities. *Person-Centered & Experiential Psychotherapies, 10*(4), 231–234. https://doi.org/10.1080/14779757.2011.626618

Proctor, G. (2017). *The dynamics of power in counselling and psychotherapy: Ethics, politics and practice*. PCCS Books.

Proctor, G. (2019). Acknowledging inequalities and meeting the unknown other: Facilitating encounter. *Person-Centered & Experiential Psychotherapies, 18*(3), 243–254. https://doi.org/10.1080/14779757.2019.1650811

Proctor, G., Cahill, J., Gore, S., Lees, J., & Shloim, N. (2021). A not-knowing, values-based and relational approach to counselling education. *British Journal of Guidance & Counselling*, 1–12. https://doi.org/10.1080/03069885.2021.1912289

Proctor, G., & Hayes, C. (2017). Counselling for depression: A response to counselling education in the twenty-first century. Ethical conflicts for a counselling approach operating within a medicalised bureaucratic health service. *British Journal of Guidance & Counselling, 45*(4), 417–426. https://doi.org/10.1080/03069885.2016.1274377

Proctor, G., McKelvie, S., Brown, M., & Cohen, S. (2020). Counsellors experiences of ethical conflicts working in IAPT. *British Journal of Guidance & Counselling*. https://doi.org/10.1080/03069885.2020.1853040

Proctor, G., Smith, L., & Akondo, D. (2021). Beyond the 'sticking plaster'? Meaningful teaching and learning about race and racism in counselling and psychotherapy training. *Psychotherapy and Politics International, 19*(2), e1580. https://doi.org/10.1002/ppi.1580

Rogers, C. R. (1959). A theory of therapy, personality, and interpersonal relationships as developed in the client-centered framework. In S. Koch (Ed.), *Psychology: A study of a science: Vol. 3. Formulations of the person and the social context* (pp. 184–256). New York: McGraw-Hill.

Rose, N. (1985). *The psychological complex*. Routledge and Kegan Paul.

Saad, L. (2020). *Me and white supremacy: How to recognise your privilege, combat racism and change the world*. Hachette UK.

Sethi, A. (2021). *I belong here: A journey along the backbone of Britain*. Bloomsbury Publishing.

Index

Note: Page numbers followed by "n" denote endnotes.

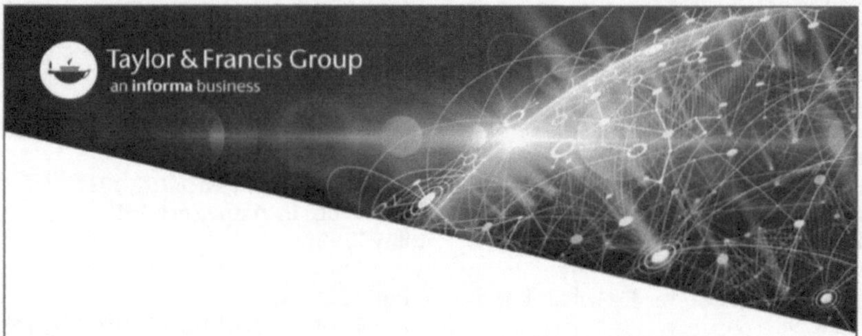